Lung Function Test

T0249742

Commissioning Editor: Laurence Hunter
Development Editor: Fiona Conn
Project Manager: Louisa Talbott
Designer/Design Direction: Stewart Larking/Mark Rogers
Illustration Manager: Jennifer Rose
Illustrator: Antbits Ltd

Lung Function Tests Made Easy

Robert J Shiner

MRCS, FRCP, FRCPC

Honorary Consultant Physician in Respiratory Medicine,
Hammersmith Hospital,
Imperial College Healthcare NHS Trust;
Honorary Senior Lecturer,
National Heart and Lung Institute,
Imperial College London
London, UK

Joerg Steier

MD(D), PhD (UK)

Consultant Physician,
Lane Fox Respiratory Unit/Sleep Disorders Centre,
Guy's & St Thomas' NHS Foundation Trust,
King's Health Partners,
London, UK

ELSEVIER
CHURCHILL
LIVINGSTONE

Edinburgh London New York Oxford Philadelphia St Louis Sydney Toronto 2013

ELSEVIER
CHURCHILL
LIVINGSTONE

© 2013 Elsevier Ltd. All rights reserved.

No part of this publication may be reproduced or transmitted in any form or by any means, electronic or mechanical, including photocopying, recording, or any information storage and retrieval system, without permission in writing from the publisher. Details on how to seek permission, further information about the Publisher's permissions policies and our arrangements with organizations such as the Copyright Clearance Center and the Copyright Licensing Agency, can be found at our website: www.elsevier.com/permissions. This book and the individual contributions contained in it are protected under copyright by the Publisher (other than as may be noted herein).

ISBN 978-0-7020-3520-3

British Library Cataloguing in Publication Data
A catalogue record for this book is available from the British Library

Library of Congress Cataloging in Publication Data
A catalog record for this book is available from the Library of Congress

Notices
Knowledge and best practice in this field are constantly changing. As new research and experience broaden our understanding, changes in research methods, professional practices, or medical treatment may become necessary.

Practitioners and researchers must always rely on their own experience and knowledge in evaluating and using any information, methods, compounds, or experiments described herein. In using such information or methods they should be mindful of their own safety and the safety of others, including parties for whom they have a professional responsibility.

With respect to any drug or pharmaceutical products identified, readers are advised to check the most current information provided (i) on procedures featured or (ii) by the manufacturer of each product to be administered, to verify the recommended dose or formula, the method and duration of administration, and contraindications. It is the responsibility of practitioners, relying on their own experience and knowledge of their patients, to make diagnoses, to determine dosages and the best treatment for each individual patient, and to take all appropriate safety precautions.

To the fullest extent of the law, neither the Publisher nor the authors, contributors, or editors, assume any liability for any injury and/or damage to persons or property as a matter of products liability, negligence or otherwise, or from any use or operation of any methods, products, instructions, or ideas contained in the material herein.

ELSEVIER your source for books, journals and multimedia in the health sciences

www.elsevierhealth.com

Working together to grow
libraries in developing countries

www.elsevier.com | www.bookaid.org | www.sabre.org

ELSEVIER   BOOK AID International   Sabre Foundation

Preface

Historically, it was always accepted that breathing was a vital function of life. Breathing was often connected to the soul, and early on in human civilisation, disordered breathing was recognised as a feature of disease. However, it was not possible to measure lung function and quantify air volume and flow properties accurately until suitable methods were developed.

Lung function testing has evolved over the years from a tool used purely for research to a commonly utilised form of clinical investigation. The importance of performing a variety of tests in patients suffering from respiratory diseases was widely accepted by specialists for many years, but more recently there has been an increase in awareness amongst additional groups of medical and paramedical personnel involved in the investigation and management of the common forms of chronic airflow obstruction (asthma and chronic obstructive pulmonary disease), as well as many forms of restrictive lung diseases. Lung volume, gas exchange abnormalities and exercise limitations are noted in a variety of pulmonary and systemic diseases, and knowledge of these may be crucial in determining management. The management algorithms in current guidelines for these disorders include lung function parameters.

The structure of this book is designed so that different chapters can be read as stand-alone sections, but cross-referencing to the other chapters completes the picture for the interested reader. It begins with lung structure and anatomy, proceeds to basic functional considerations and then moves on to discuss the tests themselves. Particular attention is given to spirometry and lung volume measurements, each of which is dealt with in a separate chapter. Following the basic principles of testing, we describe functional assessment of exercise capacity and respiratory muscle strength, and conclude with preoperative evaluation and recommendations. We have elected to devote a full chapter to preoperative evaluation, as more patients are now undergoing surgery despite various levels of respiratory insufficiency. Although thoroughly researched, in keeping with the rest of the 'Made Easy' series of books, there is no formal referencing.

Anyone using pulmonary function tests must also be aware of the limitations and technical pitfalls of this form of physiological testing. Lung function testing relies on patient compliance, 'operator' motivation, satisfactory hardware (selection, reliability and calibration of the equipment) and accurate software (as reflected in correctly predicted normal values when compared to subjects of the same population group). Faults in any of these factors can result in aberrant results. There is a wide perception that obtaining lung function results is rather like pressing the button on a console and automatically receiving a printout of the correct results and it is for that reason that we included sections in many of the chapters (and a dedicated chapter in the case of spirometry) on the pitfalls of the tests. We feel that by appreciating these limitations, clinicians will be more rigorous in their testing and more demanding of their lung function laboratories.

Boxes have been added to help emphasise important topics in the text. In addition, we have highlighted questions that can be used for short tutorials or problem-based learning. These features summarise important points that may facilitate a better understanding of the results and lead to further background reading. We have included a section on blood gas abnormalities in chapters where these are relevant to the content, but for a more comprehensive approach to blood gases and their abnormalities, we refer the reader to another book in the series, *Arterial Blood Gases Made Easy*, by I. Henessey and A. Japp (Churchill Livingstone, 2007).

Despite the fact that many departments of respiratory medicine manage patients with sleep-related problems, particularly sleep-disordered breathing, this discipline is not strictly a part of lung function testing and cannot be adequately covered in a book of this size, so we have not included it.

The book is aimed at doctors, medical students, general practitioners, nurses, inhalation therapists and those involved in clinical research or pharmaceutical studies who frequently employ physiological measurement and monitoring techniques. We have endeavoured to provide a considerable amount of basic scientific information while focusing on the practical aspects of lung function testing, as this broad audience will have a range of educational backgrounds.

Overall, we have aimed to create a book that is useful for both the interested and the occasional reader, building on basic knowledge, and helpful in the clinical setting.

RJS
JS

Acknowledgements

We would like to thank Professor J.M.B. Hughes (National Heart and Lung Institute, Imperial College School of Medicine, London, UK) for his comprehensive review and help with the manuscript.

We would sincerely like to thank our wives, Claudie and Caroline, and our families for putting up with our absences whilst we worked on the book.

Contents

Abbreviations

Abbreviation	Definition (Unit of measurement)
$AaDO_2$	Alveolo-arterial pressure gradient
AHR	Airway hyperresponsiveness
ALS	Amyotrophic lateral sclerosis; see also MND
ASA	American Society of Anesthesiologists
AT	Anaerobic threshold
ATPS	Ambient temperature, pressure and saturation
ATS	American Thoracic Society
AV	Atrio-ventricular
BAMPS	Bilateral anterolateral magnetic phrenic nerve stimulation
BE	Base excess
BMI	Body mass index (kg/m^2)
BTPS	Body temperature, pressure and fully saturated
BTS	British Thoracic Society
C	Capacitance
CABG	Coronary-arterial bypass graft
CAO	Chronic airflow obstruction
CI	Confidence interval
CMAP	Compound muscle action potential (mV)
CPET	Cardiopulmonary exercise testing
CO	Carbon monoxide
CO_2	Carbon dioxide
COPD	Chronic obstructive pulmonary disease
Cough P_{gas}	Maximal cough gastric pressure (cmH_2O)
CPAP	Continuous positive airway pressure
DLCO	Diffusion capacity for carbon monoxide (TLCO) (mmol/min/kPa)
2,3 DPG	2,3-diphosphoglycerate
ECG	Electrocardiogram
ECSC	European Coal and Steel Community
ERS	European Respiratory Society
ERV	Expiratory reserve volume (L)
ESWT	Endurance shuttle walk test
FEF	Forced expiratory flow at certain levels of vital capacity, same as MEF or $\dot{V}_{max}$ (e.g. 25%, 50%, 75% or 25–75% of FVC) (L/min)
FEV_1	Forced expiratory volume in 1 s (L)
FEV_6	Forced expiratory volume in 6 s (L)
FIF	Forced inspiratory flow, same as MIF (L/min)

FRC Functional residual capacity, derived from helium dilution method (L)

F_{res} Resonance frequency

FVC Forced vital capacity (L)

GI Gastrointestinal

GOLD Global Initiative for Obstructive Lung Disease

H^+ Proton ion

Hb Haemoglobin (g/dL)

HbF Fetal haemoglobin (g/dL)

HR Heart rate (beats per min)

I Inertance

IC Inspiratory capacity (L)

IRV Inspiratory reserve volume (L)

ISWT Incremental shuttle walk test

ITGV Intrathoracic gas volume, derived from body plethysmograph (L)

KCO Transfer coefficient (Krogh factor) for carbon monoxide (TLCO (DLCO)/VA) (mmol/min/kPa/L)

kPa Kilo Pascal (conversion factor to mmHg is multiplying by 7.5)

LABA Long-acting beta-agonists

LBBB Left bundle branch block

MEF Maximal expiratory flow at certain levels of vital capacity, same as FEF or $\dot{V}_{max}$ (e.g. 25%, 50%, 75% or 25–75% of FVC) (L/min)

MEFV Maximal expiratory flow–volume curve

MEP Maximal expiratory pressure, often referred to as PE_{max} (cmH_2O)

MET Metabolic equivalents of tasks

MIF Maximal inspiratory flow at certain levels of vital capacity, same as FIF (e.g. 50%) (L/min)

MIFV Maximal inspiratory flow–volume curve

MIP Maximal inspiratory pressure, often referred to as PI_{max} (cmH_2O)

mmHg Millimetre of mercury (conversion factor for kPa is dividing by 7.5)

MND Motor neuron disease; see also ALS

MVV Maximal voluntary ventilation (L/min)

NSCLC Non-small cell lung cancer

OR Odds ratio

OSA Obstructive sleep apnoea

O_2 Oxygen

P Pressure (cmH_2O)

$paCO_2$ Partial pressure of carbon dioxide (kPa or mmHg)

P_{alv} Pressure within alveolus

paO_2 Partial pressure of oxygen (kPa or mmHg)

P_{atm} Atmospheric pressure

P_b Bronchial pressure (cmH_2O)

PC20 Provoking concentration to reduce FEV_1 by 20%

PD20 Provoking total dose of agent to cause a fall of 20% in the FEV_1

P_{di} Transdiaphragmatic pressure (cmH_2O)

PEF Peak expiratory flow (L/min)

P_{el} Elastic recoil pressure

PE_{max} Maximal expiratory pressure, often referred to as MEP (cmH_2O)

P_{50} Partial pressure of oxygen when 50% of haemoglobin is saturated with oxygen $(mmHg)$

P_{gas} Gastric pressure (cmH_2O)

PI_{max} Maximal inspiratory pressure, often referred to as MIP (cmH_2O)

P_{mouth} Mouth pressure (cmH_2O)

P_{nasal} Nasal pressure (cmH_2O)

P_{oes} Oesophageal pressure (cmH_2O)

PPC Postoperative pulmonary complications

P_{pl} Pleural pressure (cmH_2O)

Ppo Predicted postoperative

PTCA Percutaneous transluminal coronary angioplasty

P_{tp} Transpulmonary pressure (cmH_2O)

r Radius

R Resistance

R_{aw} Airway resistance $(kPa *s/L)$

RBBB Right bundle branch block

RCRI Revised cardiac risk index

R_{osc} Resistance measured by oscillation

RQ Respiratory quotient, calculated as $\dot{V}CO_2/\dot{V}O_2$

RV Residual volume (L)

SABA Short-acting beta-agonists

SB Single breath

SCLC Small cell lung cancer

SD Standard deviation

SEVC Slow expiratory vital capacity (L)

SIVC Slow inspiratory vital capacity (L)

6-MWT 6-minute walk test

SLE Systemic lupus erythematosus

Sniff P_{di} Maximal sniff transdiaphragmatic pressure (cmH_2O)

Sniff P_{nasal} Maximal sniff nasal pressure (cmH_2O)

Sniff P_{oes} Maximal sniff oesophageal pressure (cmH_2O)

sR_{aw} Specific airway resistance $(kPa *s)$

SS Steady state

SVC Slow vital capacity (L)

TEA Thoracic epidural anaesthesia

TLC Total lung capacity (L)

TLC_B TLC as measured by the body plethysmography method (L)

TLC_{He} TLC as measured by the helium dilution method (L)

TLCO Transfer factor for carbon monoxide (DLCO) $(mmol/min/kPa)$

Twitch P_{di} Twitch transdiaphragmatic pressure, measured following magnetic or electric stimulation of the phrenic nerve (cmH_2O)

Twitch T10 Twitch gastric pressure, measured following magnetic stimulation of the 10th thoracic nerve root (cmH_2O)

UAMPS Unilateral anterolateral magnetic phrenic nerve stimulation

V Volume (L)
V_A Alveolar volume (L)
VATS Video-assisted thoracoscopic surgery
VC Vital capacity (L)
$\dot{V}CO_2$ Exhalation of carbon dioxide (L/min)
V_D Dead space volume (L)
$\dot{V}E$ Minute ventilation (L/min)

$\dot{V}E_{max}$ Maximal minute ventilation reached during exercise test (L/min)
$\dot{V}O_2$ Oxygen uptake (L/min)
$\dot{V}O_2/HR$ Oxygen pulse (L)
$\dot{V}O_{2max}$ Maximal oxygen uptake (L/min)
V_T Tidal volume (L)

W Workload (Watt)
W_{max} Maximal workload (Watt)

X Reactance

Z Impedance

CHAPTER 1

Respiratory Structure and Function

KEY POINTS

- The key functions of the respiratory system include transport of gases (oxygen and carbon dioxide) in and out of the lung, diffusion of gases into the blood, and transport of gases within the blood to and from the organs. It also fulfils a variety of other functions (e.g. cough, phonation, mucociliary clearance), which involve multiple organs.
- The respiratory system can be divided into the upper and the lower respiratory tracts separated by the glottis.
- Changes in the diameter of the upper airways have a significant and exponential (r^4) impact on the airway resistance.

INTRODUCTION

The respiratory system comprises multiple organs and fulfils very diverse functions. The most proximal parts are the upper airways, which comprise the nose, mouth, pharynx and larynx; these continue to the lower respiratory tract, which includes the trachea, bronchi, bronchioles and alveoli (Figure 1.1). Once oxygen passes beyond the basal membrane of the lung (air–blood barrier), the capillaries, arteries, veins and blood containing haemoglobin play an important role in gas exchange and gas transport. Similarly, the tissue surrounding the lung, which includes pleura, chest and neuromuscular system, forms the respiratory muscle pump, essential for respiratory function. All the organs mentioned above play a key role in at least one of the three basic functions of the respiratory system (Figure 1.2):

1. Ventilation
2. Diffusion
3. Perfusion.

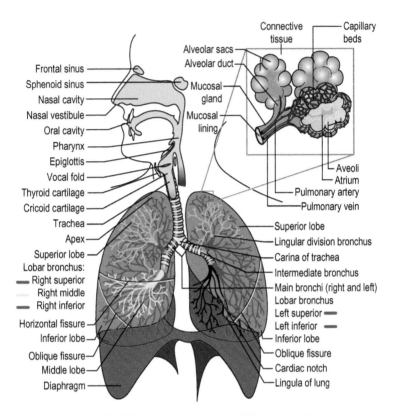

Fig. 1.1 The respiratory system, including upper and lower respiratory tracts and diaphragm. The magnified inset top right shows the alveoli surrounded by capillaries.

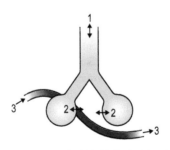

Fig. 1.2 Schematic illustration of the vital functions of the respiratory system. 1. Ventilation. 2. Diffusion. 3. Perfusion.

Each of these three functions can lead to disease if it fails in the respective organ. Ventilation, perfusion and diffusion have to be synchronised to provide optimal control of breathing. Asynchrony may cause ventilation–perfusion mismatch or impaired control of breathing.

As well as being instrumental in oxygen (O_2) uptake and carbon dioxide (CO_2) elimination, the respiratory system plays an important role in acid–base homeostasis, speech, defecation and micturition. It is also at the forefront of host defence and allergy exposure, and has a participating role in sensing taste and smell. Air inhaled through the nose is filtered, humidified and warmed. The larynx and epiglottis stop food and liquids entering our lower respiratory tract (see Figure 1.1).

STRUCTURE OF THE RESPIRATORY SYSTEM

The anatomy of the respiratory system can be divided into several functional parts and organs. The conducting airway consists of the upper airway (from nose/mouth to the larynx), trachea and main bronchi (with a diameter of around 2 cm in an adult), further dividing into the segmental bronchi and, finally, the terminal bronchioles (with a diameter of less than 2 mm). The gas exchange region of the lung includes the respiratory bronchioles and alveolar ducts, as well as the alveolar sacs. Surrounding the lung is the pleura, which has a visceral and a parietal part. The chest wall and the spinal column shape the thorax. The respiratory muscles pump air into the lung; expiration is passive at rest but can be enforced during exercise or when needed, using the expiratory muscles (mainly abdominal). The respiratory muscle pump is innervated and its function closely monitored by the central nervous system and the brain stem via several afferent and efferent nerves and feedback mechanisms (chemo- and baroreceptors). The phrenic nerve is worth mentioning here as it leaves the spine between the 3rd and 5th cervical segments (C3–C5) bilaterally and runs through the mediastinum to both hemi-diaphragms, activating the strongest inspiratory muscle, the diaphragm (Figure 1.3; Chapter 7).

In the air-conducting zone of the respiratory system diseases are usually caused by obstruction of the airway, which diminishes the overall cross-sectional area (Figure 1.10); this leads to an increased resistance and in some

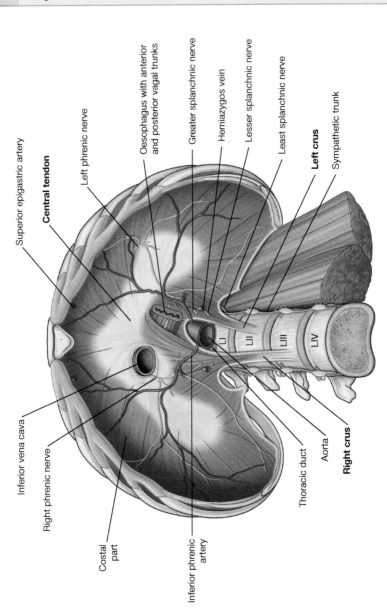

Fig. 1.3 The human diaphragm, view from the abdominal cavity
(From Drake R et al. Gray's anatomy for students. Edinburgh: Churchill Livingstone, 2009 with permission.)

cases to total airway occlusion. The impact of the airway diameter on ventilation is demonstrated by Equation 1.1:

EQ Equation 1.1

Modified Poiseuille's Equation

$$\dot{V} = \frac{\Delta P \cdot \pi r^4}{8\eta \cdot L}$$

ΔP = pressure change, L = length of the airway, η = viscosity of the gas, $\dot{V}$ = ventilation, r = radius of the airway.

Minute ventilation is directly influenced by the work of breathing (ΔP), the airway geometry (radius and length) and the consistency of the inhaled gas (viscosity). Change of the radius (r^4) has the greatest impact: an increase of 10% in the radius of the airway would result in an overall rise of 46% in ventilation, while narrowing the airway by 10% of the radius would lead to a 44% reduction of ventilation, assuming that all other parameters remained the same and work of breathing did not increase.

Narrowed airways may lead to an increase in work of breathing and, as a result of turbulent airflow, stridor may be observed. Stridor is generally distinguished as inspiratory or expiratory, and in clinical practice this distinction may yield information about the location of the airway obstruction. Inspiratory stridor is typically caused by an extrathoracic airway problem (Chapter 3). A physiological phenomenon, the Bernoulli's principle, may even lead to a total collapse of the extrathoracic airway in inspiration, while the intrathoracic airways are usually widened in inspiration due to the expansion of the chest, with the resulting negative pleural pressure transmitting the force to the lung parenchyma and bronchi. In contrast, expiratory stridor may be a sign of intrathoracic tracheal or bronchial obstruction as the intrathoracic airways collapse with a decrease in lung volume and the extrathoracic airways are kept open by gas escaping from the chest.

Potential factors causing proximal (upper) airway obstruction include various kinds of external compressive obstruction, teeth, tongue and mandible, tonsils, epiglottis, retropharyngeal space, soft palate, vocal cords and subglottic trachea (Figures 1.4 and 1.5).

Factors leading to subglottic airway obstruction are tracheomalacia and tracheal stenosis, frequently observed following intubation trauma or abnormal high cuff pressure, use of an endotracheal tube, intratracheal mass and extrinsic compression by mediastinal structures (vascular, adenopathy, tumour/goitre).

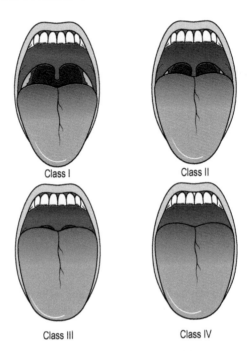

Class I   Class II

Class III   Class IV

Fig. 1.4 Schematic view of the oral cavity. The Mallampati index is a simple scoring system for pharyngeal obstruction and a narrowed upper airway due to cranio-facial shape, tongue size and obesity. It is used to assess potential difficulties during intubation and correlates with obstructive sleep apnoea.

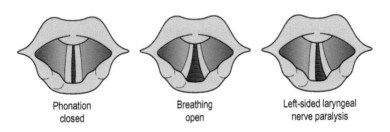

Phonation   Breathing   Left-sided laryngeal
closed   open   nerve paralysis

Fig. 1.5 Schematic illustration of the vocal cords. This is the view seen by an investigator standing behind the patient's head and looking into the upper airway, e.g. during intubation.

Trachea and Main Bronchi

The diameter of the trachea is shaped like a horseshoe, with a rigid, U-shaped cartilaginous anterior part and a posterior membrane separating it from the oesophagus. The trachea splits into the left and the right main bronchi at the bifurcation, also called the carina. This area is important for the cough reflex, as it contains a network of tactile, sensitive receptors. The main bronchi enter the lungs at their respective hilus. Like the trachea, they are protected by cartilage (Figure 1.6).

Bronchi and Lung

The main bronchi lead to the lobular bronchi, which consist of the upper, middle and lower lobes on the right, and the upper (including the lingula) and lower lobes on the left (Figure 1.1). The next generation of airways is made up of the segmental and subsegmental bronchi. The right side of the lung has ten different segments: three in the upper lobe, two in the middle lobe and five in the lower lobe. The left side contains of nine segments: five in the upper lobe, two of which are in the lingula and four in the lower lobe. The missing segment is number 7, which is considered to be left out due to the heart taking up its space. The anatomy is important in certain clinical scenarios, e.g. to manœuvre a bronchoscope, to identify locations on a chest X-ray or CT scan of the thorax, and to make decisions

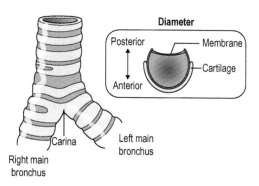

Fig. 1.6 Schematic illustration of the trachea and main bronchi. The right main stem is at a steeper angle than the left main bronchus; it is also wider and shorter. Aspiration of foreign bodies is therefore more likely to occur into the right main bronchus.

before lung resections. The bronchi further divide (there are 23 generations over-all) until, most proximally, the air reaches the alveolar sacs for the purpose of gas exchange.

Alveoli

The respiratory bronchioles lead to the alveolar ducts. The ducts are further con-nected to the alveolar sacs containing the alveoli, grouped around the ducts like grapes. The basic gas exchange unit is called the acinus. The interior surface of the alveoli produces surfactant to reduce surface tension. The exterior alveolus is covered with fine capillaries, separated from the air only by a thin layer of epithe-lium, basal membrane and endothelium (Figures 1.1 and 6.3; Chapter 6) of around $1\,\mu m$, through which gases diffuse according to their partial pressure gradient. The overall surface area of all the alveoli available for the gas exchange process is approximately $140\ m^2$.

Pleura

The pleura forms a thin layer that covers the outside of the lung, the inside of the chest, the upper part of the diaphragm and the mediastinum. It is separated into visceral and parietal sections. In contrast to the lung parenchyma, the pleura is very sensitive and pain can be caused by irritation during acute diseases of the chest. There is a small gap between the parietal and visceral parts, which is filled with fluid; the lung can slide along the inner surface of the chest and still remain expanded because of the sealed pleural space. The pleural pressure is usually neg-ative or subatmospheric, and is determined by the elasticity of the lung and the chest wall, which oppose each other (see compliance, Chapter 2). However, if the pleura is damaged and air enters the pleural space, the elastic recoil of the lung becomes unopposed and the lung collapses, causing a pneumothorax. The pleura usually balances production and reabsorption of fluid but, in disease, production can be increased or reabsorption can be impaired, leading to fluid collection in the pleural space and a pleural effusion.

Chest Wall and Respiratory Muscles

The respiratory muscles are an important part of the respiratory system, as the muscle pump is responsible for ventilating air into and, if required, out of the chest. All the muscles involved in respiration insert on to the skeletal structures of the chest (vertebrae, ribs, shoulder blades, clavicles and sternum). They provide the lung with protection and stability, but leave enough space for expansion while breathing and moving. Failure of the respiratory muscle pump commonly results in hypercapnic respiratory failure (type II), which is characterised by an increase in CO_2 levels, accompanied by low oxygen levels (see Chapters 6 and 7).

Respiratory muscles can be broadly distinguished by inspiratory and expiratory function; some, like the diaphragm, work constantly in inspiration, while other accessory muscle groups can be recruited when demanded. In normal subjects, the scalene, sternocleidomastoid, parasternal and external intercostal muscles can contribute to inspiration (in addition to the diaphragm), even during quiet breathing, and this effect is more pronounced during more active breathing manœuvres. Quiet expiration in normal subjects is predominantly the result of passive elastic recoil of the lung and chest wall. The main expiratory muscles, the rectus abdominis and external oblique, tend to contribute to expiration only during exercise and forced breathing manœuvres.

During rapid-eye-movement (REM) sleep, however, the diaphragm is usually the only inspiratory skeletal muscle active, as the other skeletal muscles undergo a functional atonia. Therefore, REM sleep-related hypoventilation may occur should the diaphragm (Figure 1.3) become weak or paralysed. Other inspiratory or accessory respiratory muscles are in the neck (scalene, sternocleidomastoid, trapezius), shoulders and intercostals (parasternal, internal and external; Chapter 7). Expiratory muscles are predominantly composed of the abdominal muscles and intercostals. They can be recruited during forced expiration, during exercise or in disease but are inactive at rest in healthy subjects. Problems affecting the respiratory muscle pump may be of neural or muscular origin, or may be caused by neuromuscular junction abnormalities. The central nervous system with its neural respiratory motor output is responsible for modifying our breathing pattern and the control of breathing (Figure 1.7).

FUNCTIONS OF THE RESPIRATORY SYSTEM

The central function of the respiratory system is gas exchange. The body requires oxygen for energy and metabolic function; in addition, the carbon dioxide produced during these processes needs to be eliminated by ventilation. For this purpose, neural respiratory drive activates the respiratory muscle pump, which contracts and creates a negative intrathoracic pressure during inspiration. The diaphragm descends and the chest wall muscles help to widen the thorax.

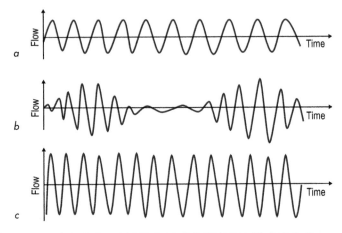

Fig. 1.7 *Schematic illustration of different breathing patterns.* **(a)** *Normal quiet breathing;* **(b)** *Cheyne–Stokes respiration (e.g. in heart failure or due to medication) with periodic crescendo–decrescendo pattern and apnoeas;* **(c)** *Kussmaul breathing (e.g. in metabolic acidosis) with respiratory rate and depth increased.*

Air entry follows the pressure gradient through the upper airway into the chest. Simultaneously, the cardiac pump provides blood for oxygenation and to eliminate CO_2, distributing the oxygenated blood throughout the body.

There is a marked interdependence between respiratory and cardiac systems. Chemoreceptors, particularly within the carotid and aortic bodies, detect changes in oxygen and H^+-ions in the blood. Reduced oxygen content leads to a reflex increase in pulmonary ventilation and systemic arterial blood pressure. Baroreceptors sense changes in the systemic arterial blood pressure and provoke a compensatory adjustment of the heart rate and systemic vascular resistance. The Euler–Liljestrand effect, also called hypoxic vasoconstriction, regulates pulmonary vascular resistance to avoid ventilation–perfusion mismatch in the lung.

Ventilation–Perfusion

In normal adult subjects, ventilation takes place at approximately 5–8 L/min. At the same time, cardiac output is around 5–6 L/min. In this case, the blood flow matches the gas flow almost 1:1, although gravity favours better perfusion in the lower lobes of the lung in the upright subject, while the upper lobes are usually

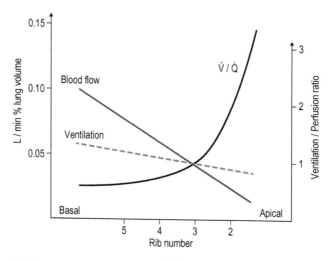

Fig. 1.8 *Schematic Ventilation/Perfusion (V̇/Q̇) ratio of the lung, upright. The base of the lung is well perfused, while the apex is relatively better ventilated, resulting in a decreasing V̇/Q̇ ratio from top to bottom.*

slightly better ventilated (Figure 1.8). Minute ventilation can be varied in many ways, e.g. due to rib cage displacement, frequency or tidal volume. Inspiration requires actively recruiting respiratory muscle, while expiration usually follows passively due to the elastic recoil.

 Why is it important that Ventilation matches Perfusion?

Let us assume that all ventilation went to the right lung and all circulation to the left lung, gas exchange would not be possible; a sensible adjustment between ventilation and perfusion is therefore crucial for successful gas exchange. *Ideally*, ventilation and perfusion must be *exactly* matched; ventilation must be distributed to perfused areas and perfusion must be distributed to ventilated areas.

Ventilation–perfusion inequality is the most common cause of arterial hypoxaemia (Figure 1.9). Gas exchange abnormalities are mainly due to mismatching between ventilation and blood flow in the lungs, and less often caused by alveolar hypoventilation, right-to-left shunts and diffusion defects.

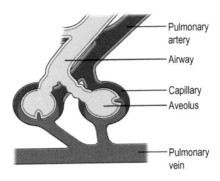

Pulmonary artery

Airway

Capillary

Aveolus

Pulmonary vein

Fig. 1.9 *Ventilation–Perfusion relationship in the alveoli and capillaries. (From Cherniack R. Pulmonary function testing. Philadelphia: WB Saunders, 1977 with permission)*

Cross-Sectional Area of the Airways

The total cross-sectional area of the airway increases with each new airway generation, of which there are a total of 23. The velocity of gas during inspiration exponentially decreases from the upper airway towards the level of the respiratory bronchiole. At this level, diffusion (Chapter 6) becomes the predominant mode of ventilation (Figure 1.10).

Dead Space/V_D

Dead space is defined as the volume of inspired air that is not participating in gas exchange. It can be separated into an anatomical and a physiological dead space.

The anatomical dead space includes the air in the nose, mouth, pharynx, trachea, bronchi and bronchioles. It amounts to approximately 150 mL at rest and makes up around 20–30% of the tidal volume. It is decreased by jaw depression and neck flexion.

The physiological dead space is the total amount of inspired air that is not participating in gas exchange, including that in the anatomical dead space. In addition to the latter, it includes parts of the lung that are ventilated but not perfused appropriately. If the physiological dead space is increased, this may result in significantly less effective minute ventilation.

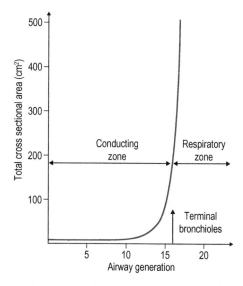

Fig. 1.10 *Schematic illustration of the total cross-sectional area (CSA) of the airways. As the inspired air enters the lower airways, the overall CSA increases and conduction velocity decreases. Once the air enters the respiratory zone, the main mode of transportation is diffusion (see Chapter 6).*

What happens when the tidal volume is low in a ventilated patient?

It is important to consider the dead space in a ventilated patient. A low tidal volume combined with a high respiratory rate may significantly ventilate dead space but may not provide gas (oxygen) that reaches the alveolar space and participates in gas exchange.

Safeguarding the Airway

To secure airway patency it is sometimes necessary to safeguard the airway. The safest option, although it is invasive, is the use of an endotracheal tube, which can be inserted via the nose or the mouth. It may be necessary to use sedation and neuromuscular blockade to place the tube successfully. However, endotracheal tubes elongate and narrow the airway (Equation 1.1).

In certain conditions, a surgical airway via tracheotomy may be necessary in the management of a patient. This has the advantage of reducing anatomic dead space by as much as 60% which is often indicated in patients who need prolonged periods of invasive ventilation.

Mucociliary Clearance

The inner surface of the respiratory system is covered with ciliated epithelium, which produces mucus. There is a directed and synchronised movement of the cilia, transporting mucus, dust or small foreign bodies towards the pharynx, where they can be swallowed. This mucociliary clearance efficiently clears the tracheo-bronchial tree of particles between 2 and 10 μm in diameter. Larger particles (> 10 μm) are usually filtered in the nose; although the nose is lined with the same epithelium, the upper airways are usually cleared by sneezing, coughing and sniffing. Inhaled particles of less than 2 μm may reach the alveolar ducts and sac, where there are no cilia and, therefore, expulsion is poor. The particle size is important to consider once medication is inhaled or nebulised, as only fine droplets will pass the nose and continue to be deposited in the smaller airways.

? What happens when clearance of the airways is impaired?

Mucociliary clearance is an important issue because many diseases are caused by an insufficient clearance mechanism; this may be due to thick secretions with a high viscosity (e.g. cystic fibrosis), or reduced mobility of the cilia on the inner surfaces of the respiratory system (e.g. genetic mutations causing ciliary dysfunction). Longstanding mucoid impaction may lead to bronchiectasis, colonisation with pathogenic organisms (frequently *Pseudomonas*) and severe lower respiratory tract infection (e.g. pneumonia).

Transport of Gases in the Blood

Ventilation and perfusion eventually provide oxygen (O_2) to the cells and eliminate carbon dioxide (CO_2). Efficient transport of O_2 and CO_2 in the blood depend on several factors (Chapter 6):

1. the properties of haemoglobin
2. the physical chemistry of the blood
3. regulation of the systemic arterial circulation, which is required to maintain optimal respiratory gas tensions in the tissue.

SUMMARY

The respiratory system requires a range of organs to function and work in synchrony, specifically the pulmonary, cardiac, haematological and neuromuscular systems. It is vital for normal respiratory function that ventilation, diffusion and perfusion are closely linked. Airway diameter is the predominant geometric determinant when considering airflow. Stridor, especially inspiratory, is a hallmark feature of upper airway obstruction. Many conditions may result in upper airway obstruction but the immediate therapy is always the same: control of the airway.

CHAPTER 2

Mechanics of Breathing

KEY POINTS

- In normal resting subjects, inspiration is actively supported by respiratory muscle activity, and expiration happens passively due to elastic recoil of the respiratory system.
- Both lung and chest wall compliance vary in various respiratory disorders and contribute significantly to the work of breathing.
- Surfactant acts to stabilise the lungs and can markedly decrease the surface tension of the air–liquid interface.
- Two major components, elastic and flow-resistive forces, contribute to the work of breathing and may be altered in disease states.

INTRODUCTION

Breathing is partly active and partly passive. Usually, in order to expand the chest adequately during inspiration, the respiratory muscles (Chapter 7) need to generate enough force to overcome the resistance created by the respiratory apparatus and gas in the respiratory tract. When the respiratory muscles start to relax, expiration follows, usually passively due to the elastic retraction of the lung and the chest wall. However, with relaxation of the respiratory muscles, as occurs at the end of a normal expiration, there is a volume of air left in the lungs: the functional residual capacity (FRC; Figure 3.1). The FRC level is determined by the balance of elastic forces exerted by the lungs and chest wall. When expiration is actively supported, additional volume (expiratory reserve volume, ERV; Figure 3.1) may be recruited, e.g. during exercise.

What is elasticity?

Elasticity is defined as the property of matter that causes it to return to its resting shape after deformation by an external force.

The lung typically tends to collapse due to elastic properties, but this is opposed by the force from the chest wall holding the lungs in place with adhesive forces via the pleural gap. However, if the chest is opened, e.g. injury, accident or iatrogenic, and air enters the pleural gap the lung collapses.

Two factors are responsible for this phenomenon:

1. Connective tissues, elastin and collagen in lung
2. Surface tension generated in the alveoli.

What is the pleural pressure (P_{pl})?

The pleural pressure represents the force that is generated by the chest wall to keep the lung from collapse due to elastic recoil. It is usually negative at rest and varies with the breathing pattern. A surrogate marker for the pleural pressure is the oesophageal pressure, which is often used for clinical measurements as it is easier to access via an oesophageal catheter than measuring the pleural pressure invasively.

Changes in the oesophageal pressure follow changes in the pleural pressure because its walls are thin and have little tone. Pressures are the driving forces for movement of the chest and airflow (Figure 2.1).

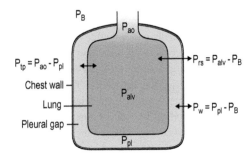

Fig. 2.1 *Schematic illustration of the respiratory system and its pressures. P_{alv} = alveolar pressure; P_{ao} = pressure at airway opening; P_B = barometric pressure; P_{pl} = pleural pressure; P_{rs} = pressure of the respiratory system; P_{tp} = transpulmonary pressure; P_w = pressure across the chest wall.*

Transpulmonary Pressure (P_{tp})

The transpulmonary pressure is defined as the pressure difference between airway opening and pleural space (P_{ao}-P_{pl}; Figure 2.1). It is an important marker for the compliance of the lung and can be used to derive the pressure–volume curve determining elastic properties of the lung.

 What is compliance?

$$c = \Delta V / \Delta P$$

Compliance (c) is defined as the change of volume (ΔV) per change of pressure (ΔP). It defines the characteristics of the entire respiratory apparatus (or the chest wall/lungs) when calculated across each part of the respiratory system (lung, chest wall or both; Figure 2.1).

STATIC COMPLIANCE IN DIFFERENT CONDITIONS

The static inspiratory and expiratory pressure–volume relationship provides useful information about the elasticity of the lung. It can be plotted by measuring transpulmonary pressure (P_{tp}; Figure 2.1) between total lung capacity (TLC) and residual volume (RV, Chapter 5).

Here are some examples of how static compliance may change with the underlying condition (c, Figure 2.2):

- In healthy lungs, the application of a pressure of $5 cmH_2O$ results in an inflation of 1 litre of air:

  $c = 1 L/5 cmH_2O = 0.20 L/cmH_2O$

- In emphysema, the application of a pressure of $5 cmH_2O$ results in an inflation of 2 litres of air because of loss of elastic recoil:

  $c = 2 L/5 cmH_2O = 0.40 L/cmH_2O$

- In pulmonary fibrosis, due to an increase in elastic recoil, the application of a pressure of $5 cmH_2O$ results in an inflation of only 0.5 litre of air:

  $c = 0.5 L/5 cmH_2O = 0.10 L/cmH_2O$

Approximately half of the elastic recoil of the lung comes from the elastic properties of its tissue, just as there is recoil in an inflated rubber balloon. The other half of the elastic recoil of the lungs is generated from the unique

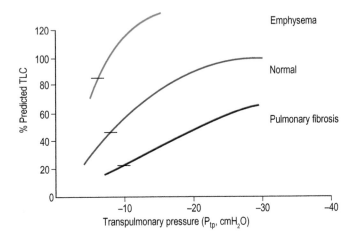

Fig. 2.2 *Schematic Pressure (P$_{tp}$)–Volume (% predicted TLC) curve in normal subjects and patients with emphysema and pulmonary fibrosis. There is a disease-specific difference, with a low slope in fibrosis and a high slope in emphysema, representing low and high compliance (c = ΔV/ΔP).*

structure of millions of alveoli, which are filled with liquid and connected to the atmospheric pressure via the bronchial tree.

Filling the lung with saline neutralises the effect of the surface tension and elastic recoil in the alveoli, shifting the compliance curve to the left and abolishing the difference that is usually observed between the inspiratory and expiratory portions of the compliance curve; this is known as hysteresis (Figure 2.3).

The elastic forces of the lungs and those of the chest wall vary at different lung volumes, but different types of compliance must be recognised:

1. Compliance of the chest wall
2. Compliance of the lung
3. Combined compliance of the chest wall–lung system (c$_{total}$).

This distinction becomes more obvious when the relaxation pressure curve is considered. The relaxation pressure curve summarises the total compliance curve of the respiratory system (c$_{total}$, Figure 2.4). At FRC level, the forces exerted by the lung and the chest wall are equal but pulling in opposite directions. Therefore the relaxation pressure is '0' or atmospheric. Above FRC level, the resulting

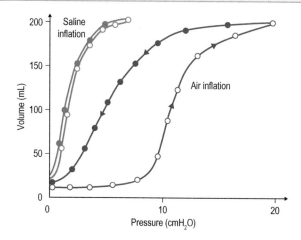

Fig. 2.3 *Pressure–Volume plot with air (red slope) and saline (green slope) inflation, inspiratory (open circles) and expiratory (solid circles) slopes. The effect of hysteresis with the loss of difference between inspiratory and expiratory slopes can be recognised by the left shift of the trace.*

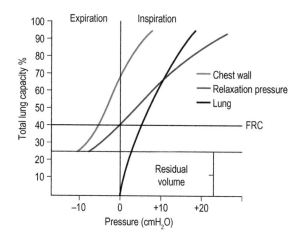

Fig. 2.4 *Relationship between the elastic forces of the lungs and chest wall at different lung volumes. The relaxation pressure is the sum of the chest wall and the lung pressures. This means that the relaxation pressure is '0' where chest wall and lung pressures are of equal value but opposite in direction; this is the case at FRC.*

relaxation pressure is positive. Below FRC, the chest wall is pulling towards inspiration (expansion), relatively more so than the lungs are pulling in an expiratory direction (deflation). This results in a negative relaxation pressure.

In contrast to static compliance, which is obtained by plotting transpulmonary pressure against lung volume when there is no airflow, dynamic compliance is determined during spontaneous breathing. Dynamic compliance is defined as the volume change during a breath divided by the change in oesophageal or pleural pressure between end-expiration and end-inspiration. It is a less reliable measurement than static compliance and will also depend on the lung volume at which the subject is breathing. However, it is easier to measure in clinical practice, as static compliance with an accurate measurement of chest wall recoil is difficult to obtain. Factors such as age, obesity and chest wall deformities (e.g. ankylosing spondylitis, kyphoscoliosis) should be considered when measuring compliance, as they may cause a stiffening of the chest wall.

ELASTIC RESISTANCE/ELASTANCE

Elastic resistance is defined as the reciprocal of compliance. It indicates pressure change per unit of volume change, while the compliance is defined as change in volume per unit of pressure change. To understand the basic principle of compliance and elastic resistance, it is helpful to imagine a simple spring:

- When a spring is easy to distend, it has a low elastic resistance but a high compliance.
- When a spring is hard to distend, it has a high elastic resistance but a low compliance.

Which factors stabilise the lungs?

Surfactant (Surface Active Agent)
Surfactant can markedly decrease the surface tension of an air–liquid interface. It forms relatively late in gestation and can be assessed in amniotic fluid; it is deficient in conditions such as respiratory distress syndrome (RDS).

Interdependence of Lung Units
Adjacent alveoli share a single common wall. In this system, the tendency of one alveolus or lung unit to collapse is opposed by the support of surrounding units.

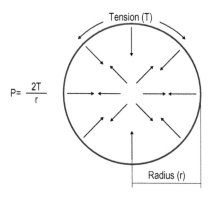

Fig. 2.5 *Law of Laplace, determining the pressure in the alveoli, which prevents a collapse to a lower volume. P = pressure (the transmural pressure necessary to keep a spherical bubble of liquid inflated to a fixed size); T = tension in the wall; r = radius of the bubble.*

There is a tendency for the lung to reduce in volume due to the elasticity of the lung parenchyma and the surface tension at the alveolar air–liquid barrier (Figure 2.5).

Surface tension is dynamically altered and closely tuned to the alveolar radius. It is reduced with expiratory decrease of the alveolar radius, and increases with the next inspiratory expansion. Therefore, according to the law of Laplace, surfactant is necessary to keep the alveolar pressure (P) constant throughout the ventilatory cycle. Without surfactant, smaller alveoli would empty their content into larger ones and collapse if the wall tension did not decrease.

AIRWAY RESISTANCE

In addition to the elastic recoil of the lungs and the chest wall, the respiratory muscles encounter flow-resistive properties during inspiratory activity. The force generation that must be applied during inspiration depends on the amount of resistance to airflow.

Resistance to flow is produced by the upper airways and the tracheo-bronchial tree and is due to the frictional resistance of tissues sliding over each other in the

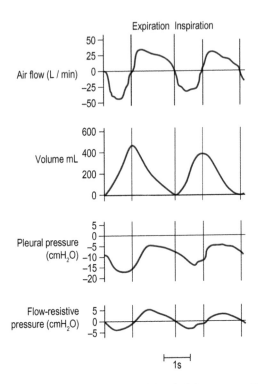

Fig. 2.6 *Relationship between airflow, tidal volume, pleural pressure and flow-resistive pressure during resting breathing.*

lung parenchyma and chest wall. At end-inspiration and end-expiration there is no airflow, and the flow-resistive pressure is atmospheric (Figure 2.6). During expiration the flow-resistive pressure is higher than during inspiration. Compliance can be calculated by dividing the volume change between these two points by the change in pleural pressure.

The total pressure in the pleural space during breathing (P_{tp}) is the sum of that required to overcome elastic resistance (P_{el}) and flow resistance (P_r, Figure 2.7a).

Flow resistance is approximately $1–3\,cmH_2O/L/s$ but can be increased 10–15-fold with airflow obstruction, as observed in asthma or chronic obstructive pulmonary disease (COPD).

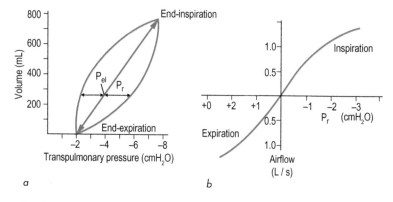

Fig. 2.7 Pressure–volume and flow–pressure curves. **(a)** The determination of flow resistance from the relationship between volume and transpulmonary pressure (P_{tp}). P_{el} (the pressure required to overcome elastic resistance) is derived by a line joining end-inspiration and end-expiration. P_r is the pressure required to overcome flow resistance; $P_r = P_{tp} - P_{el}$; **(b)** Pressure–airflow plot of P_r against airflow; in this case, P_r can be derived from the slope of the linear portion of the curve ($\Delta P_r / \Delta$airflow).

Airway resistance is derived from flow resistance per airflow (P_r/airflow ($\dot{V}$)), and the pressure required to overcome flow resistance (P_r) can be derived from the slope of the pressure–flow plot at the linear part of the curve ($\Delta P_r / \Delta$airflow, Figure 2.7b). The relationship between pressure change and airflow is due to laminar resistance but the deviation from the straight line signifies a disproportionate increase in the pressure required to produce a further increase in airflow due to turbulent resistance.

 How do we draw air into our lungs?

Air enters and leaves the lungs due to changes in the intrathoracic pressure following a negative pressure gradient in inspiration and positive pressure in expiration. By increasing the size of the thorax, the inspiratory muscles lower intrathoracic pressure relative to atmospheric pressure, causing bulk flow into the airways.

What happens during a forced expiration to the airways?

The positive intrathoracic pressure causes dynamic compression of the airways.

DYNAMIC AIRWAY COMPRESSION DURING FORCED EXPIRATION

Once maximal airflow ($\dot{V}_{max}$) has been achieved during forced expiration, the resistance to airflow must rise in direct proportion to the driving pressure. The rise in airflow resistance that occurs at each lung volume is due to the dynamic compression of the airways. Elastic recoil (P_{el}) helps oppose dynamic compression by traction on the small airways, and the alveolar P_{el} becomes the driving pressure for continued airflow (Figure 2.8). During expiration the pressure in the airways drops from the alveolus (P_{alv}) to the mouth ($P_{atmospheric}$).

The equal pressure point (EPP, 'choke point') is the point at which intrabronchial and extrabronchial pressures are equal. Further upstream from the EPP (towards the mouth) there is a transmural pressure that tends to narrow or close the airway. Flow limitation occurs at specific sites of narrowing ('choke points') along the airway and these 'choke points' are likely to form at locations where the transmural pressures become negative (Figure 2.8).

When dynamic compression of the airways occurs, the maximum driving force for flow will become the difference between alveolar pressure (P_{alv}) and the intrapleural pressure (P_{pl}); this is not determined by effort but by the volume and compliance of the lung (Equation 2.1; Chapter 3).

EQ Equation 2.1

Lung Elastic Recoil Pressure

$$P_{el} = P_{alv} - P_{pl}$$

P_{alv} = alveolar pressure; P_{el} = lung elastic recoil pressure; P_{pl} = pleural pressure

During dynamic compression of the airways in forced expiration, the flow-limiting site is typically in second and third generations of airways. Greater effort (increased P_{pl}) results in greater compression with decreased radius.

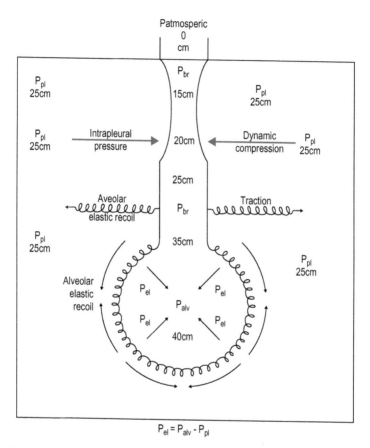

Fig. 2.8 Relationship between changes in atmospheric ($P_{atmospheric}$), pleural (P_{pl}), bronchial (P_{br}), alveolar (P_{alv}) and elastic recoil (P_{el}) pressures during a forced expiration. Pressures are reported in cmH_2O.

The compression starts at EPP (Figure 2.8) in the cartilage-free airways within the lung. In disease, the weakened airways can actually collapse, causing air to become trapped behind the blockade. Pursed lips breathing moves the EPP to the mouth, bringing relief to the patient with airway obstruction (see resistance, Chapter 1).

27

What happens as lung volume decreases?

The change in recoil with decreased lung volume is significant, airways narrow, airway resistance increases and the flow-limiting site moves more peripherally. Thus, in late forced expiration, flow is increasingly determined by the properties of the small peripheral airways (Figures 2.9 and 2.10).

At high lung volume, maximum expiratory flow rises with increasing effort, while at lower lung volumes increasing pressure raises the airflow rate to a maximum and further effort produces no further increase in flow; this is thought to be a result of airway compression and increased resistance. The airways are more distended at higher lung volumes because the transpulmonary pressure is greater, so that flow resistance is lower (Figure 2.11).

Of similar importance to airway resistance is the airway calibre, as this increases with lung volume. In addition, regional airway resistance decreases as a function of airway generation (Figure 2.12).

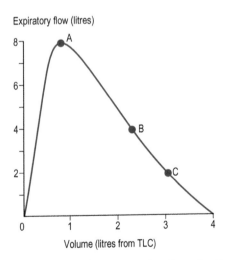

Fig. 2.9 *Flow–Volume plot in a normal subject, indicating three different levels of lung volume from which the plots in Figure 2.10 are derived.*

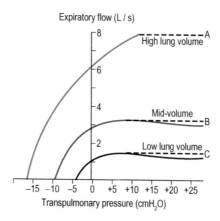

Fig. 2.10 Isovolume pressure–flow curve obtained in a normal subject at three levels of lung inflation. **(A)** The effort-dependent part of the forced expiratory manœuvre is shown at a high lung volume; **(B** and **C)** The effort-independent portion is shown at mid-volume and low lung volume.

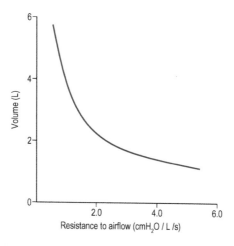

Fig. 2.11 Relationship between lung volume and resistance to airflow in a normal subject. The airways are wider at a higher lung volume, creating a low flow resistance; at low lung volumes, the airways narrow down and reach the so-called 'closing volume', and consequently resistance increases.

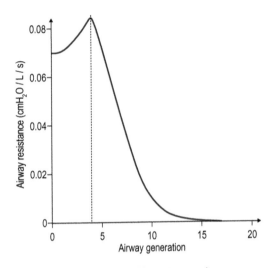

Fig. 2.12 *The relationship between airway generation and airway resistance.*

The highest regional resistance is at airway generation 4, which represents medium-sized bronchi of short length; here, frequent branching results in highly non-laminar airflow with extreme turbulence (Figures 2.12 and 2.13).

Large airways with a diameter of > 2 mm frequently develop a disorganised turbulent airflow pattern. This is characterised by a high Reynolds number (Re) of > 2000 (Equation 2.2).

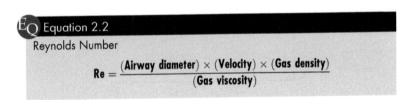

Equation 2.2

Reynolds Number

$$Re = \frac{(\text{Airway diameter}) \times (\text{Velocity}) \times (\text{Gas density})}{(\text{Gas viscosity})}$$

Turbulent flow may, however, extend more distally with airway pathology. Gas density can be reduced by breathing different gases, e.g. helium, and this approach can be useful when treating airflow obstruction, particularly of the upper airway (Equation 2.2).

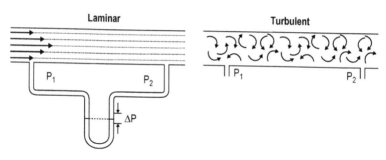

Fig. 2.13 *Schematic representation of the two types of airflow profile: laminar (small airways) and turbulent (large airways). P is the pressure and ΔP the pressure gradient between P_1 and P_2.*

Small airways with a diameter of < 2 mm develop a smooth regular laminar airflow pattern like a series of concentric tubes sliding past each other. They have a low Reynold's Number (Re < 2000). However, laminar flow follows Poiseuille's equation (Equation 1.1). This means that, for a given pressure gradient, doubling the length of the tube will cause a reduced flow rate of 50%, and reducing the tube diameter by 50% will decrease the flow 16-fold under laminar flow conditions.

Airway resistance is also influenced by the phase of respiration, as it is lower in inspiration than in expiration. Vagal and sympathetic tone may similarly modify resistance in disease, although little resting vagal or sympathetic tone is found under normal conditions.

Blood gases may also influence airway resistance; hypocapnia, if severe enough, can cause bronchoconstriction. Hypercapnia, however, has no known effect on airway resistance.

WORK OF BREATHING

 What is work of breathing?

The work of breathing is the work required by the respiratory muscles in order to overcome the mechanical impedance to respiration caused by the lung, chest wall and abdominal contents during breathing. It is the sum of the work required to overcome both elastic properties and flow resistance.

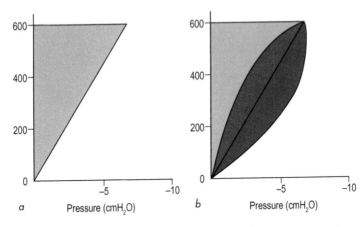

Fig. 2.14 A plot of tidal volume against pleural pressure. **(a)** The shaded portion represents the mechanical work of breathing necessary to overcome elastic resistance; **(b)** An additional shaded envelope has been added (in red) which represents the work of breathing required to overcome flow resistance.

To consider the work of breathing it is useful to calculate the product of pressure and volume. In expiration, the two shaded areas overlap, indicating that expiration is passive as a result of the elastic force of the lung that developed during inspiration (Figure 2.14). In inspiration, the total work of breathing performed is the sum of the elastic work and that is required to overcome inspiratory flow resistance. About two-thirds of the work is developed against elastic forces.

Although expiration is usually passive, during forced expiration, or even during tidal breathing in a patient suffering from airway disease, additional expiratory mechanical work may be required. In asthma, there is an increase in flow-resistive work as a result of the airway narrowing. In that situation, the elastic energy stored during inspiration will not produce enough airflow during expiration and the expiratory muscles must cope with an increased load and perform extra work (Figure 2.15).

In pulmonary fibrosis the work required to overcome the flow resistance of the stiff lungs is similar to that in healthy subjects, but more work is required to overcome the increased elastic resistance of the 'stiff lungs' (Figure 2.16).

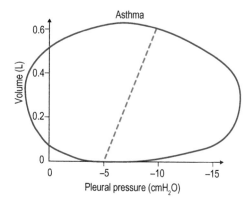

Fig. 2.15 Mechanical work of breathing during tidal breathing in a patient suffering from asthma. The flow-resistive loop falls outside the area of elastic work (compare to Figure 2.14a) requiring additional activity of the respiratory muscle pump in expiration.

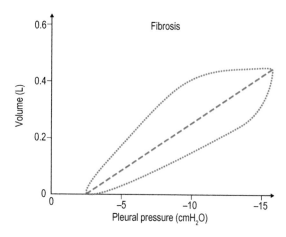

Fig. 2.16 Mechanical work of breathing during tidal breathing in a patient suffering from pulmonary fibrosis. (See also Figure 2.14)

Mechanical Work and Alveolar Ventilation

Work of breathing can affect the pattern of breathing and therefore the amount of ventilation available for gas exchange. For any given alveolar ventilation there is an optimal respiratory rate and tidal volume, i.e. the most 'economical' or 'value-for-money', at which point the total mechanical work of breathing is minimal (Figure 2.17).

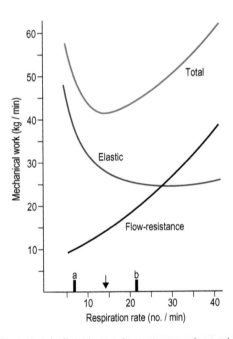

Fig. 2.17 *Mechanical work of breathing and respiratory rate during tidal breathing in a healthy person. The optimal respiratory rate in a healthy person is indicated by the arrow. Should the respiratory rate be reduced to less than optimal (a), then the flow-resistive work will decrease but the amount of work to overcome elastic resistance will increase. When the respiratory rate is higher than optimal (b), then, in order for the same alveolar ventilation to be maintained, total mechanical work must increase as the flow resistance will increase.*

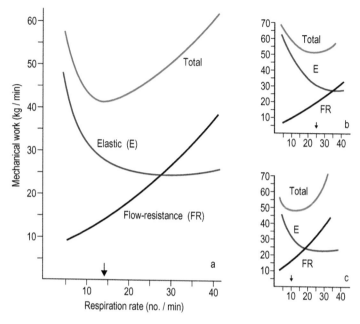

Fig. 2.18 Effect of respiratory rate on the mechanical work of breathing.
(a) In normal subjects; (b) When the elastic work (E) is increased, e.g. in pulmonary fibrosis; (c) When the non-elastic or flow-resistive (FR) work is increased, e.g. in asthma.

When the mechanical properties of the respiratory apparatus are altered by disease, the respiratory pattern is often altered accordingly. Elastic resistance is increased in pulmonary fibrosis and the curve describing the relationship between respiratory rate and mechanical work required to overcome elastic resistance is shifted upward and to the right. Therefore, as the work is minimal at increased frequency, respiration becomes rapid and shallow (Figure 2.18b). With bronchial obstruction, such as in asthma, flow resistance is increased and the curve representing the relationship between respiratory rate and mechanical work required to overcome flow resistance is shifted upward and to the left. The work is minimal at a lower frequency, and in this situation respiration becomes slower and deeper (Figure 2.18c).

35

SUMMARY

Compliance of the lung and the chest wall can profoundly alter lung mechanics and breathing pattern. Lung stability relies on the interdependence of lung units and on surfactant, which can decrease the surface tension of the air–liquid interface. The total pressure in the pleural space developed by the respiratory muscles is the sum of the pressure required to overcome elastic forces and flow resistance. Airflow resistance in the airways is influenced by multiple factors, such as lung volume, airway diameter, gas density and flow velocity. The work of breathing is different in airway disorders, pulmonary fibrosis and chest wall abnormalities and requires adjusting for frequency and volume in order to be optimised.

CHAPTER 3

Spirometry

KEY POINTS

- Peak flow measurement and spirometry are basic and easily available tests of lung function.
- Spirometry measures static (volume) and dynamic (flow) parameters.
- PEF, FEV_1, FVC and VC are the most important spirometric parameters that indicate obstructive or restrictive disease.
- Spirometry is an important tool in the diagnosis, management and follow-up of respiratory disorders.
- Tests of airway hyperresponsiveness and bronchodilatation using spirometric monitoring are a useful diagnostic tool for asthma.

INTRODUCTION

Spirometry facilitates the measurement of airflow and lung volumes (Box 3.1). It allows for volume assessment measured at the mouth and, together with lung volume measurement (Chapter 5), gives a comprehensive evaluation of all lung compartments. Static (volume) and dynamic (flow = volume over time) parameters are assessed using standard spirometry manœuvres (Figure 3.1). It is an uncomplicated investigation and the equipment required (spirometer; Figure 3.2) is affordable and usually available in a chest unit and in many community-based primary and secondary care clinics. However, it is a volitional test of flow and volumes, and thus is directly dependent on the motivation of the patient and the experience of the staff.

METHODS AND MEASUREMENTS

Spirometry is often the first pulmonary function test performed on patients with suspected pulmonary disease, as it can be helpful in screening.

There are different ways to measure flow and volume. One is actually to measure the volume in a calibrated chamber, as is used in a bellows spirometer

Box 3.1 Clinical indications for spirometry

- Assessment of symptoms of pulmonary diseases, dyspnoea, orthopnoea, cough, wheezing, etc.
- Follow-up of pulmonary disease
- Monitoring of disease progress and assessment of treatment effects
- Assessment of pulmonary complications of primary non-pulmonary disease (e.g. heart failure, systemic lupus erythematosus)
- Preoperative risk assessment
- Occupational health-related questions
- Rehabilitation

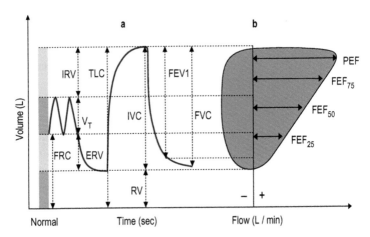

Fig. 3.1 Spirometry manœuvre. **(a)** Recording of volume over time; **(b)** Flow–volume curve. Lung volumes and expiratory flow rates of a healthy subject are visualised. ERV = expiratory reserve volume, FEF = forced expiratory flow, FEV_1 = forced expiratory volume in 1 second, FRC = functional residual capacity, FVC = forced vital capacity, IRV = inspiratory reserve volume, IVC = inspiratory vital capacity, PEF = peak expiratory flow, RV = residual volume, TLC = total lung capacity, V_T = tidal volume. PEF is dependent on effort and it therefore reflects flow in the large airways. The mid-expiratory flow as reflected in the FEF_{25-75}, is relatively effort-independent and mainly reflects flow in the small airways.

(Figure 3.2). Another method is to use a pneumotachograph (Figure 3.3) and this is most often done in conjunction with electronic spirometers. The pneumotachograph measures the proportional pressure gradient over a defined resistance, which can be used to calculate the flow according to Ohm's law (Equation 3.1).

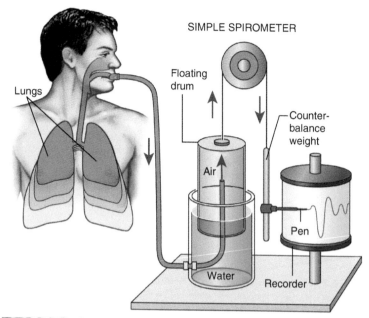

SIMPLE SPIROMETER

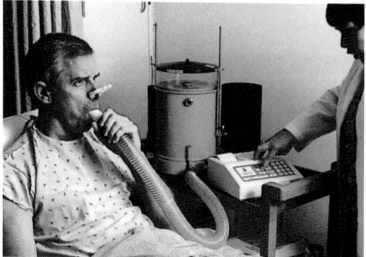

Fig. 3.2 *Examples of spirometers.* **(a)** *Classic spirometer design showing how the volume of air exhaled and inhaled is recorded as a rising and falling line;* **(b)** *A simple spirometer attached to a computerised recording device. Flow is derived from volume over time.*

(From Patton K, Thibodeau G. Anatomy and physiology. St Louis: Mosby, 2010 with permission)

Pneumotachograph

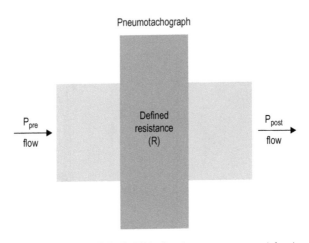

Fig. 3.3 *Schematic pneumotachograph. Airflow has to overcome a defined resistance (R). Using the pressure gradient (ΔP = P_{pre} − P_{post}), the flow can be calculated according to Ohm's law.*

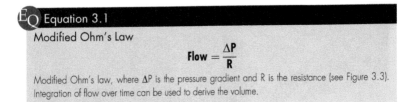

Equation 3.1

Modified Ohm's Law

$$\text{Flow} = \frac{\Delta P}{R}$$

Modified Ohm's law, where ΔP is the pressure gradient and R is the resistance (see Figure 3.3). Integration of flow over time can be used to derive the volume.

Following full inflation of the chest and full expiration, the volume that can be measured at the mouth is known as the vital capacity (VC). VC includes the expiratory reserve volume (ERV) but not residual volume (RV), which is the volume in the lungs remaining after a full expiration (Figure 3.1).

This VC manœuvre normally lasts between 4 and 6 s in normal subjects but is prolonged in airway obstruction. It can be performed rapidly as a forced vital capacity (FVC) manœuvre (Figure 3.1), or as a slow vital capacity (SVC). In normal subjects the values of SVC and FVC should be very similar.

The more classical spirometers measure exhaled volume over a period of time and are displayed in that format (Figure 3.1A). The information that can be obtained from the manœuvre is the total forced volume expired (FVC) and the forced expiratory volume in the first second (FEV_1); in addition, flow (flow = volume / time) can be calculated at any point on the volume–time curve. In other words, flow can be measured from the curve between 25% and 75% of the FVC (forced expiratory flow, FEF_{25-75}, see Figure 3.1B), and at various individual places on the curve such as at 50% and 25% of FVC (FEF_{50} and FEF_{25}).

IMPORTANT PARAMETERS

Peak Flow (PEF)

The peak flow describes the maximal expiratory flow rate that can be achieved early in the expiratory manœuvre. It is a reliable test that is best assessed from a peak flow meter (Figure 3.4). The peak flow is expressed in litres/minute and percentage predicted when age, gender, height and ethnicity are considered.

Appropriate and effective asthma treament is reflected in both an improvement in absolute PEF values and a marked reduction in diurnal variability (Figure 3.5). Diurnal variation of peak flow is characterised by a morning 'dip' in

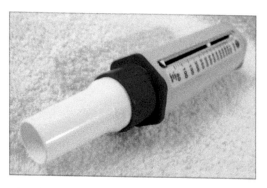

Fig. 3.4 Peak flow meter.

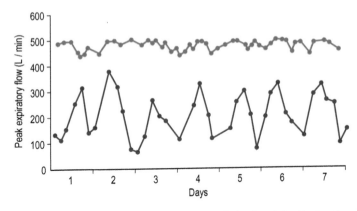

Fig. 3.5 *Diurnal peak flow variability in an uncontrolled asthmatic (red line) and response to treatment (green line).*

PEF, which is exaggerated in unstable asthma. The peak flow can be calculated either from the flow–volume curve (Figure 3.1b) or from a 'stand-alone' peak flow meter (Figure 3.4), but not from most volume spirometers (Figure 3.2a), as their response times tend to be slow and will not detect the highest flow portion of the forced expiratory manœuvre.

Forced Expiration Manœuvre

The manœuvre of maximal expiration that follows a deep breath aimed at completely filling the lungs results in the application of force to the thoracic cavity and its contents (Chapter 2). As a result, gas is expelled from the lungs as both pleural (P_{pl}) and alveolar (P_{alv}) pressures increase. This may lead to complications in airway disease, as the bronchi may collapse (Figure 3.6).

 What would happen if one drew too forcefully on a soggy straw?

The pressure inside the straw would become negative with respect to ambient pressure and the straw would collapse. At that point, no amount of additional effort would cause the flow to increase. However, if water were slowly drawn through the straw, then flow limitation might not occur.

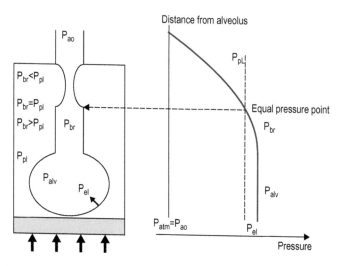

Fig. 3.6 *Dynamic compression during a forced expiration manoeuvre. P_{alv} = pressure within the alveolus, P_{atm} = atmospheric pressure, P_{br} = intrabronchial pressure, P_{el} = elastic recoil pressure of the lung, P_{ao} = pressure at airway opening, P_{pl} = pleural pressure. Thick arrows indicate the force from the respiratory muscle pump.*

? What happens when dynamic compression of the airways occurs?

The maximum driving force for flow will be the difference between alveolar pressure (P_{alv}) and intrapleural pressure (P_{pl}); it is not determined by effort but rather by the volume and compliance of the lung.

Forced Expiratory Volume in 1 Second (FEV₁)

The FEV_1 is the expired volume during the first second of a maximal expiration (Figure 3.7). It is a useful measurement that correlates well with the prognosis in asthma and chronic obstructive pulmonary disease (COPD) and declines with age and, more rapidly, in smokers. FEV_1 is expressed in litres and percentage predicted when age, gender, height and ethnicity are considered.

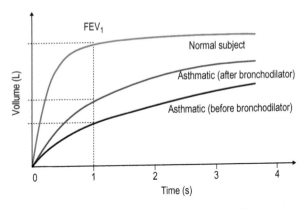

Fig. 3.7 *Three Volume–Time (V–T) curves. Curves are presented for a normal subject (green line), an asthmatic patient with bronchoconstriction prior to bronchodilator (blue line) and the same patient following bronchodilator administration (red line). The asthmatic (before bronchodilator) curve is consistent with a significant degree of airway obstruction and the value of the FEV1 can be read off the y-axis (volume) at 1 s, as indicated by the horizontal bars.*

Slow Exhaled Vital Capacity (SVC)

The SVC is defined as maximum (total) volume of air expired during a slow manœuvre from total lung capacity (TLC). It will be reduced, relative to FEV_1 (i.e. percent predicted value for SVC will be significantly less than the percent predicted value for FEV_1) in restrictive disorders. In the context of a pure restrictive disorder with no obstructive element (in practical terms, no scalloping of the flow– volume curve, normal or increased FEV_1/FVC ratio and normal mid-expiratory flow at low lung volumes), SVC is an accurate way to assess lung volumes, particularly on a longitudinal basis. In obstructive disease, slow expiration allows the patient to breathe out without airway collapse; measurement of the slow vital capacity may therefore better reflect vital capacity than a forced expiratory manœuvre (FVC).

However, if a restrictive disorder has a coexisting obstructive element, e.g. in sarcoidosis, then TLC is a more accurate way to assess and follow up the patient. The reason for this is that an increase in RV in an obstructive disorder would decrease the value of the SVC (Figure 3.8; Chapter 5). SVC is expressed in litres and percentage predicted when age, gender, height and ethnicity are considered.

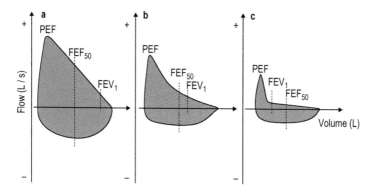

Fig. 3.8 *Three schematic Flow–Volume (F–V) curves.* **(a)** *Normal subject;* **(b)** *Patient with moderate airway obstruction;* **(c)** *Patient with severe chronic airflow obstruction.* FEV_1, FEV_1/FVC *ratio and maximal flow at 50% of the FVC* (FEF_{50}) *are diminished in airway obstruction. The F–V curve has the advantage of displaying both forced expiration and forced inspiration on the same plot. In addition, there is an element of 'pattern recognition' when considering the flow–volume curve compared to the volume–time curve.*

Forced Vital Capacity (FVC)

This is the maximum (total) volume of air measured at the mouth, either expired or inspired during a forced maximal manœuvre (Figure 3.1). The FVC may be significantly less than SVC if air trapping occurs during a forced expiratory manœuvre (Figure 3.6 and Chapter 5). It is expressed in litres and percentage predicted when age, gender, height and ethnicity are considered.

Forced Expiratory Volume in 6 Seconds (FEV₆)

The FEV_6, which measures the volume of air that can be expired in 6 seconds, is roughly equivalent to FVC in normal people. In the case of very severe airflow obstruction, exhalation may take up to 15 seconds or longer and the patient may well stop beforehand; this may result in an underestimation of the degree of airflow obstruction. The ratio of FEV_1/FEV_6 has been validated as a parameter to assess airway obstruction.

Δ SVC–FVC

The difference between slow and forced vital capacity should be minimal in normal subjects but increases with more severe chronic airflow obstruction due to increased air trapping with forced expiration (Figure 3.6).

FEV$_1$/SVC

This ratio reflects the percentage of the total volume of exhaled air that is exhaled in 1 second and was first described by Tiffeneau in 1947 (Tiffeneau Index). Values of less than 70% are indicative of airway obstruction. As FEV$_1$/SVC (or FEV$_1$/FVC) is a ratio, it has the advantage of being independent of height, gender and ethnicity, but does decrease with age due to loss of elastic recoil pressure.

FEV$_1$/FVC

This ratio is frequently used (e.g. in Global Initiative for Obstructive Lung Disease (GOLD) guidelines for COPD) instead of SVC, as it is easy to obtain from a forced expiratory manœuvre without performing an additional slow vital capacity manœuvre. However, it may also significantly underestimate the degree of obstruction when compared to FEV$_1$/SVC in obstructive disease in the presence of an increased residual volume (Figures 3.1 and 3.8; Chapter 5).

Inspiratory Capacity (IC)

The IC is measured by an inspiration to full lung inflation (TLC) from relaxed end-expiratory tidal breathing. It combines the tidal volume and inspiratory reserve volume (Figure 3.1). A reduced IC correlates well with mortality in obstructive lung disease. It can be recorded during exercise testing to determine the degree of dynamic hyperinflation.

Measures of Reduced Flow at Low Lung Volumes

In contrast to the FEV$_1$, forced expiratory parameters obtained at lower lung volumes are physiological markers of small airway (airway diameter < 2 mm) pathology. They are expressed in litres/second and percentage predicted when age, gender, height and ethnicity are considered.

FEF_{25-75}

This reflects the FEF between 25% and 75% of expired vital capacity (Figure 3.1).

FEF_{75}, FEF_{50}, FEF_{25}

These parameters describe the FEF at 75%, 50% and 25% of the FVC (Figure 3.1).

FEF_{25} is less reliable and less reproducible than FEF_{25-75} or FEF_{50}. All of these measurements are occasionally abbreviated as maximal expiratory flow (MEF), forced expiratory flow (FEF) or $\dot{V}_{max}$, which may be used as equivalents.

DIFFERENT SPIROMETRY FINDINGS IN RESPIRATORY DISEASES

What can we learn from spirometry in chronic airflow obstruction?

PEF measurements are of limited value in the diagnosis of chronic airflow obstruction but may be useful in monitoring in asthma. Therefore, in the presence of symptoms that include cough, wheeze, sputum expectoration and dyspnoea, as well as a history of atopy or exposure to risk factors such as tobacco, occupation, indoor or outdoor pollution, spirometry is mandatory to confirm the clinical diagnosis (Table 3.1).

An obstructive ventilatory defect is a disproportionate reduction of maximal airflow in relation to the maximal volume measured at the mouth (VC) that can be displaced from the lung. It is defined by a reduced FEV_1/VC ratio below the 5th percentile of the predicted value (where VC is highest when compared to FVC or SVC). If the ratio is not reduced, the shape of the flow–volume curve should

Table 3.1 Degree of airway obstruction based on the FEV_1 and FEV_1/FVC (according to GOLD Guidelines)

Degree of Severity	FEV_1 (% Predicted)	FEV_1/FVC
Mild Stage I	≥ 80	$< 70\%$
Moderate Stage II	50–79	$< 70\%$
Severe Stage III	30–49	$< 70\%$
Very Severe Stage IV	< 30 or chronic respiratory failure	$< 70\%$

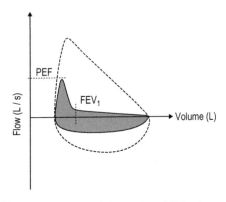

Fig. 3.9 *Flow–Volume curve in a patient with emphysema. This illustrates how the PEF is relatively better 'preserved' than the FEV_1 in severe chronic airflow obstruction (predicted Flow–Volume curve – dotted line).*

nevertheless be examined, as a 'scalloped' appearance may hint at obstructive pathology in the presence of an increased residual volume (Figure 3.9; see also Figures 3.1 and 3.8). Parameters such as IC correlate with prognosis from heart as well as lung disease, even in non-smokers, particularly as part of the IC/TLC ratio (Chapter 5).

Airflow generates resistance; in healthy adults approximately 50% of the total airway resistance is generated between the nose and the larynx, 35% of the resistance derives from the trachea and bronchi, and around 15% of the total resistance is created distal to the bronchioles (small airways).

The bronchioles do not contribute much to the total airway resistance in normal adult lungs, but this is different in infants and children. In healthy adults the total cross-sectional area of the small airways is greater than the total cross-sectional area of the central airways. In disease, small airways can therefore contribute disproportionately to the increase in total airway resistance, particularly in infants and children.

What can we learn from spirometry in restrictive disorders?

Restrictive disease is associated with reduced lung volumes. However, a reduced VC alone does not prove a restrictive defect. It may be suggestive of lung restriction when FEV_1/VC is normal or increased but, in addition, a low TLC measurement is needed to confirm the diagnosis. However, a low VC in the presence of a 'non-scalloped' or convex shape of the flow–volume loop may be supportive of the diagnosis.

Restrictive disorders may be divided into 'pulmonary' causes, such as the interstitial lung diseases, various cardiac pathologies like congestive heart failure, and 'extrapulmonary' causes, which may affect the chest wall or pleura or be neuromuscular in origin (see Chapter 5).

Unfortunately, with the exception of the measurement of seated and recumbent VC (which may be useful in neuromuscular disorders), further lung function tests (particularly gas exchange measurements) are required to differentiate between the above categories of restrictive disorders (see Chapters 5 and 6).

In addition, VC is normally measured when seated. A fall in VC of less than 15% when the subject changes from a seated to a supine posture has been demonstrated in normal subjects. However, a reliable and reproducible measurement of a decrease of more than 15% in VC with change of posture is suggestive of significant diaphragmatic weakness or paralysis; if it is reduced by more than 30%, it is suggestive of bilateral diaphragmatic weakness or paralysis.

Upper Airway Obstruction

Spirometry is usually performed following inflation to TLC and then rapid expiration to the end of VC. At the point of end-expiration a rapid inspiration can be achieved and recorded as the inspiratory portion of the flow–volume curve (Figure 3.10). In chronic airflow obstruction the inspiratory limitation is less than the expiratory, this difference being most pronounced in the more severely obstructed (Figure 3.9).

Obstruction in the upper airways can, if there is at least a 50% obstruction, be detected from forced inspiratory manœuvres, whereas obstruction in the lower airways can be detected from a forced expiratory manœuvre.

There are three classic patterns of flow–volume loop contours in patients with upper airway obstruction (Figure 3.10), depending on the location of the obstruction and whether the obstruction is fixed or variable.

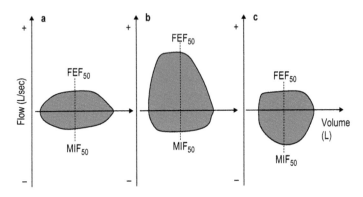

Fig. 3.10 Three patterns of maximum inspiratory flow–volume curve (MIFV) and forced expiratory flow–volume curve (MEFV) in upper airway obstruction. **(a)** Fixed intra- or extrathoracic obstruction; **(b)** Variable extrathoracic obstruction; **(c)** Variable intrathoracic obstruction. FEF_{50} = forced expiratory flow at 50% of vital capacity, MIF_{50} = maximal inspiratory flow at 50% of vital capacity.

Fixed Lesions

A fixed lesion results in a constant rate of airflow during both inspiration and expiration, as the calibre of the airway is fixed. This fixed lesion may be intra- or extrathoracic; both types result in a similar flattened flow–volume curve, in inspiration and in expiration. This pattern may be seen in post-intubation strictures, goitres and tracheal tumours (Figure 3.10a).

Variable Extrathoracic Lesions

These obstructions are different from fixed obstructions, in that they may result in changes in airway calibre, which will vary during inspiration and expiration. With variable extrathoracic obstruction, there is a characteristic pattern of obstruction above the thoracic inlet. Forced inspiration will result in a decrease in intraluminal pressure relative to the atmospheric pressure. The result is a flattening of the inspiratory limb on the maximal inspiratory flow–volume curve (MIFV). During expiration the extrathoracic airway is expandable (albeit somewhat narrowed) and the maximal expiratory flow–volume curve (MEFV) is closer to normal. This pattern may be seen in strictures of the glottis, tumours and vocal cord paralysis (Figure 3.10b).

Variable Intrathoracic Obstruction

During a forced inspiration, the pressure within the bronchus is higher than the pleural pressure outside the airways; the airways are therefore subjected to a large distending force, which results in high inspiratory flows. During expiration, compression subsequent to an increase in pleural pressures results in a decrease in the size of the airway lumen at the site of intrathoracic obstruction, producing a flattening of the expiratory limb of the flow–volume loop. This pattern is seen with variable intrathoracic lesions such as malignant tumors and tracheomalacia (Figure 3.10c).

Bronchodilator Response

Most asthmatic and some COPD patients will have a history of a significant clinical response to a short-acting bronchodilator (SABA). This can often, but not always, be reproduced by demonstrating a significant physiological response to a SABA at a particular time or on a particular day of testing in terms of an improvement in PEF, FEV_1 or FVC.

Frequently in clinical practice, a good clinical history will be the only way of diagnosing childhood asthma but the problem with having no objective physiological measurement is that severity may be more difficult to assess and treatment harder to monitor.

If physiological testing is undertaken either in children or in adults, a 'one-off' lack of response may not exclude a bronchodilator response; it should be noted that, in moderate to severe chronic airflow obstruction, bronchodilator responsiveness is a continuous variable.

It should also be noted that, if the spirometric values are good, i.e. close to normal predicted values, then a significant bronchodilator response (of $> 12\%$ in FEV_1) cannot be present; some form of provocation test will frequently be needed, particularly if the clinical diagnosis of asthma is in doubt.

Methods of Bronchodilator Response

Depending on the severity of their condition, patients are instructed to try to withhold SABAs for at least 8 hours, long-acting beta-agonists for at least 12 hours, and oral bronchodilators for 24 hours before testing. Commonly, the SABA used for assessing bronchodilator response is the short-acting beta$_2$-adrenergic receptor agonist, salbutamol (albuterol), but the addition of an inhaled short-acting anticholinergic drug might be useful in demonstrating reversibility, particularly in COPD. Salbutamol is administered either as four separate doses of 100 µg, given by metered dose inhaler using a spacer, or nebulised 5 mg salbutamol together with 2.5 mL of saline. Spirometry is performed prior to and 15 minutes following bronchodilator administration. Several criteria have been used by various global (The Global Initiative for Chronic Obstructive Lung Disease (GOLD)), European (European Respiratory Society), US (American Thoracic Society) and UK (British Thoracic Society/Scottish Intercollegiate Guidelines Network) groups to define a significant bronchodilator response.

The absolute percentage improvement and predicted percentage improvement are used as criteria for a significant response, but they fail to take proper account of how good or how poor the lung function is at the outset ('A small amount of money to a poor man is of more value than the same amount of money given to a rich man'; Figure 3.11).

FEV_1 Response

A reasonable consensus approach might be that a significant bronchodilator response in chronic airflow obstruction could be taken as an improvement in FEV_1 of at least 200 mL. This is commonly seen in asthmatics and some COPD

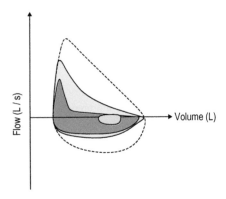

Fig. 3.11 Flow–volume curves in a patient with chronic airflow obstruction before (dark pink) and after (light pink) bronchodilator administration. Dotted lines indicate the flow–volume curve of a normal subject; the blue area shows the Flow–Volume curve during tidal breathing.

patients but an absolute improvement in FEV_1 of > 400 mL in response to a beta$_2$-adrenergic receptor agonist would be highly suggestive of a diagnosis of asthma.

 Why test for an FEV$_1$ bronchodilator response in chronic airflow obstruction?

Asthma

An FEV_1 bronchodilator response confirms the clinical diagnosis, particularly if FEV_1 response to a SABA is > 400 mL.

COPD

Testing accurately defines the post-bronchodilator FEV_1, which is highly correlated between visits and therefore a better guide to subsequent disease progression than the pre-bronchodilator value.

A response might also help to determine those patients in whom airflow obstruction is improved by this treatment.

In contrast to asthma, as many as 75% of COPD patients will not have a significant FEV_1 response but nevertheless do have an FVC response to an inhaled SABA of at least 400 mL. This fits the clinical scenario in which many COPD patients report symptomatic and functional improvement when using these drugs, despite showing little post-bronchodilator change in FEV_1. A response in terms of an increase in FVC or VC is a reflection of reduced hyperinflation, i.e. a reduction in RV following SABA administration. In addition to a flow or volume response to bronchodilatation, it is possible to demonstrate both or to have no response at all.

 Why test for an FVC bronchodilator response in chronic airways obstruction?

Asthma

Improvements in FVC tend to be relatively small compared to the percentage increase in FEV_1.

COPD

The response tends to be more marked than the percentage increase in FEV_1, particularly in those patients with a low baseline FEV_1.

BRONCHIAL CHALLENGES AND AIRWAY HYPERRESPONSIVENESS

If spirometry is normal (or near-normal), then assessment of airway hyperresponsiveness (AHR) will best discriminate asthma from other causes of chronic airflow obstruction such as COPD, bronchiectasis (including cystic fibrosis), inhaled foreign body, obliterative bronchiolitis, large airway stenosis and sarcoidosis (Figure 3.12). However, in the presence of significant airflow obstruction, tests of airway responsiveness are less helpful and SABA is the preferred next step in the diagnostic algorithm.

A clinical diagnosis of asthma must be based on a good medical history. Specifically, this means a history of recurrent episodes of wheeze, cough, dyspnoea and chest tightness, which may worsen at night (possibly with associated night wakening) and in the early morning, following exposure to pets, damp, cold air, or during or following exercise. A personal history of atopy or a family history of atopy or asthma is also frequently noted. Many patients will have had a symptomatic response to SABA treatment in the past.

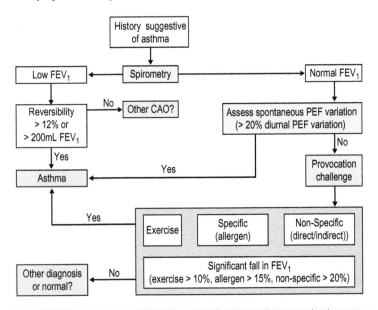

Fig. 3.12 *Schematic approach to the diagnosis of patients with suspected asthma using spirometry, bronchodilator response and provocation challenges.*

Methods of Bronchial Provocation Challenge

The principle of bronchial provocation challenges is to demonstrate AHR, as reflected in a significant reduction in FEV_1 when exposed to various agents in a population with suspected asthma (Figure 3.12).

One of the clinical characteristics of asthma is AHR, which might manifest itself as shortness of breath accompanied by wheezing or cough when exposed to cold air, exercise and allergen. In clinical practice, some tests of AHR can be useful to establish the diagnosis when there is no airway obstruction that reverses significantly following bronchodilator administration.

Specific Bronchial Provocation Challenge

Allergen challenge requires controlled inhalation of an environmental aero-allergen to which an individual is suspected to be sensitive (positive skin-prick test). Allergen inhalation challenge in sensitised subjects typically induces an early asthmatic response (EAR), with a reduction in FEV_1 of at least 15%, which is maximal within 30 minutes but resolves within 180 minutes (3 hours). Up to 50% of these responders will also experience a second delayed late asthmatic response (LAR), with a late phase of bronchoconstriction (again with a reduction in FEV_1 of at least 15%), leading to the dual asthmatic reaction (DAR; Figure 3.13). The allergen-induced LAR is

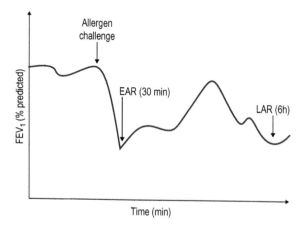

Fig. 3.13 *Allergen challenge and FEV_1 response with early (EAR) and late (LAR) schematic asthma response. The latter can occur several hours following allergen exposure.*

55

associated with airway eosinophilia. These tests are not routinely performed in most institutions and necessitate strict longer-term monitoring, often within the framework of an overnight hospital admission as a precaution against the late response (in some instances exceeding 6 hours) that may occur in some patients.

Non-specific Bronchial Provocation Challenge

The stimuli used to measure airway responsiveness can be differentiated into direct and indirect types.

Direct stimuli (histamine, methacholine) act directly on receptors of the airway smooth muscle and are most commonly used in the evaluation of adults with suspected asthma.

Indirect stimuli act through one or more intermediate pathways, most commonly via release of mediators from inflammatory cells such as mast cells. They include physical (exercise, hyperventilation, cold air, non-isotonic aerosols) and certain chemical stimuli (adenosine-5-monophosphate (AMP), mannitol; Table 3.2). It may be that the indirect stimuli are indeed more clinically relevant,

Table 3.2 Inhaled substances used for assessing non-specific airway hyperresponsiveness (Bronchial Provocation Challenge)

Type	Examples
Physical	Cold air
	Exercise
Physico-chemical	Hypertonic saline
	Water
Chemical	SO_2
	KCL
Pharmacological	Direct
	Methacholine
	Histamine
	Indirect
	AMP (adenosine-5-monophosphate)
	Mannitol
	Bradykinin
	Leukotrienes
	Carbachol
	Propranolol
	Lysine aspirin
	Sodium metabisulphite

as naturally occurring asthma is associated with symptoms on exposure to indirect-acting stimuli. In fact, indirect AHR does appear to correlate better with asthma disease activity and with airway inflammation.

In clinical practice, when evaluating the possibility of asthma, particularly in non-exercising adults, most specialists will first perform a *direct* non-specific bronchial provocation test using either histamine or methacholine. Methacholine is currently used more commonly than histamine in provocation challenges, as the latter may be associated with more systemic side effects, particularly headache, flushing and hoarseness. There is also some doubt regarding the reproducibility of AHR with histamine. These tests are very sensitive, though not entirely specific, for asthma. In other words, a diagnosis of asthma would be less likely in the presence of a negative histamine or methacholine provocation test.

The usefulness of these tests is influenced by the degree of clinical suspicion of asthma. In the presence of a reasonable degree of suspicion, this test can be very informative as a diagnostic tool but can also characterise the severity of the AHR: the lower the dose that causes a 20% fall in FEV_1 the more severe the AHR. There are various potential factors that are associated with a positive methacholine challenge test in patients without clinical asthma; these include seasonal variability, allergy (allergic and non-allergic rhinitis), respiratory infection (particularly viral croup, sinusitis, mycoplasma), smoking, chemical irritants, cardiovascular conditions (mitral valve stenosis, congestive heart failure), gastrointestinal disorders (Crohn's disease, ulcerative colitis, gastro-oesophageal reflux), autoimmune disorders (rheumatoid arthritis, Sjögren's syndrome), sarcoidosis or being an athlete.

A negative direct non-specific provocation test should be followed by an indirect non-specific provocation test, such as exercise, AMP or mannitol in order to exclude AHR.

Direct Provocation Challenge

A number of different protocols have been used to perform and interpret methacholine challenge tests. The principle is to inhale a quantity of a provoking agent and then perform an FEV_1 manœuvre. If there is a reduction of less than 20%, the dose is increased and the FEV_1 manœuvre repeated; it is repeated incrementally, until either a 20% reduction in FEV_1 is observed or the inhaled dose is so high that significant AHR has effectively been excluded. Non-asthmatic patients might also demonstrate some degree of bronchoconstriction when inhaling methacholine or histamine, but only at much higher doses (Table 3.2, Figure 3.14).

Prior to the test, bronchodilators should be withheld for up to 48 hours if possible (depending on whether they are short-acting or long-acting), as should leukotriene antagonists, antihistamines and glucocorticoids. Coffee, tea, cola drinks and chocolate should also be withheld on the day of the study.

The three most commonly performed protocols are as follows:

1. 2-minute tidal breathing via a nebuliser for each dose, followed by an FEV_1 measurement before proceeding to a higher dose
2. a five-breath dosimeter technique in which the individual takes five deep breaths of methacholine (or histamine) concentration from a nebuliser, followed by an FEV_1 manœuvre before proceeding to a higher dose
3. a hand bulb nebuliser activated during inhalation (Yan protocol), which is particularly useful for epidemiological surveys.

PC_{20}

The PC_{20} is the provoking concentration of the agent that is required to induce a fall in FEV_1 of 20% or more. If the PC_{20} is < 8 mg/mL, the test result is held to indicate an asthmatic response (Figure 3.14).

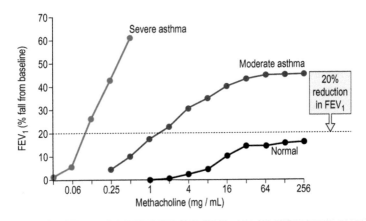

Fig. 3.14 *Methacholine provocation challenge in severe (green) and moderate (red) asthma, as well as in a normal subject (blue). The dotted line indicates PC_{20}.*

PD_{20}

The PD_{20} is the provoking total dose of the agent used during the test that was required to provoke a fall in FEV_1 of 20% or more. A PD_{20} of < 8 µmol is considered to be within the asthmatic range.

Indirect Provocation and Exercise Challenge

Bronchospasm that is induced by exercise is a frequent complaint in children and exercising young adults. Therefore it is considered by some to be an accepted first test when testing for AHR in that population. The key stimulus for the occurrence of exercise-induced bronchospasm is not the exercise itself, but rather the coinciding hyperventilation. When present, it has the advantage of being specific for asthma and effectively differentiates asthma from other forms of chronic airflow obstruction.

Potential disadvantages are that such testing is only diagnostic in about two-thirds of asthmatic patients. It may not even be present in the same asthmatic person who is tested on different occasions. Unlike in most other provocation tests, the extent of the bronchoconstrictor response cannot be strictly monitored during the tests and can be substantially more than the 20% reduction in FEV_1 considered to be a positive response to conclude other provocation tests.

The FEV_1 is measured prior to and following 6 minutes of treadmill running with the treadmill set at a slope of $10°$. The subjects run continuously at a speed of 5 km/h. FEV_1 is measured before and 3, 5 and 10 minutes after exercise. Some laboratories only measure the FEV_1 once after 10 minutes, which can be a problem in children and young adults in whom the exercise-induced decrease in FEV_1 may occur more rapidly and subsequently returns to near baseline levels well within 10 minutes. This phenomenon appears to be age-dependent; the younger the subject, the earlier the nadir of bronchoconstriction occurs – sometimes as soon as 3 minutes – following the end of exercise.

The challenge should be performed in an air-conditioned laboratory so that the subjects breathe room air at a temperature of 20–26°C and a relative humidity of 48–56%. Heart rate, which should reach 80–95% of the predicted maximum, is measured and the greatest fall in FEV_1 after exercise is calculated as a percentage of the pre-exercise value; 10% or more is considered significant. An alternative approach in children, which is less well validated but could prove to be more applicable in the community setting, would be to measure reduction in either FEV_1 or PEF prior to and following a 6-minute free-running test.

LIMITATIONS OF SPIROMETRY

Spirometry requires full inhalation to TLC and the expired volume measured at the mouth is the VC; it therefore does not include the measurement of RV that cannot be assessed directly at the mouth but nevertheless accounts for approximately 20% of the TLC in normal subjects (Figure 3.1).

The difference between the forced and slow vital capacity manœuvres, the FVC and SVC, is small in normal subjects. However, in patients with significant chronic airflow obstruction the FVC may be significantly less than the SVC, which is the result of air being trapped in the lung secondary to airway collapse. The finding of such a discrepancy in FVC and SVC should lead to additional measurements, particularly the determination of lung volumes (Figure 3.1 and Chapter 5).

The importance of measuring lung volumes as an add-on test to spirometry is well illustrated by the increase in RV noted in many patients with chronic airflow obstruction, such as asthma or COPD, and reflects the degree of air trapping. A degree of hyperinflation usually results in an increase in functional residual capacity (FRC), which is the volume of air present in the lung at normal resting end-expiration (Chapter 5).

What happens when FRC increases?

The patient tends to breathe at a higher lung volume, i.e. closer to TLC; in physiological terms, the value for the IC is reduced and the IC/TLC ratio is also reduced. This is termed hyperinflation and it is usually a result of airflow limitation. Hyperinflation acts as a compensatory mechanism. At higher lung volumes there is decreased airway resistance and increased elastic recoil, resulting in improved expiratory flow.

The spirometry trace should be free of artifacts from cough, glottis closure or suboptimal effort. The peak flow should be reached early on during the forced expiratory manœuvre, and expiration should be at least 6 s long and reach a plateau. Repeated measurements of FEV_1 and FVC should be within accepted levels of variability (Chapter 4).

SUMMARY

Spirometry is an easily available method providing the clinician with important information regarding respiratory diagnosis or the aetiology of breathlessness and airway disease. It measures dynamic and static parameters that can help diagnose obstructive or restrictive lung disease, monitor and assess treatment effect. The peak flow measurement can further assist in monitoring chronic airflow obstruction, particularly in asthmatic patients. In some cases, bronchodilator response, tests of airway hyperresponsiveness and provocation tests may be required in the diagnostic algorithm.

CHAPTER 4

Pitfalls in Spirometry

KEY POINTS

- Obtaining a reproducible, correctly performed manœuvre is crucial.
- Equipment and software-related problems are common.
- Patient- and technician-related performance is frequently suboptimal.
- Most solutions for prevention of microbial transmission are inadequate.

INTRODUCTION

In spirometry, it is important to understand the limitations of the method in order to read and interpret the data from lung function test results properly and to judge critically. The problem is that we do not exactly know how closely the value that we read off the spirometer approximates to the correct value. It may be confounded by various problems (Box 4.1).

The reasons for inter-laboratory differences are varied but include diurnal variation, inaccuracy in height measurement, variations in reference values, poor equipment maintenance and calibration, and differences in hardware and software. When individual commercially available electronic spirometers have been tested by independent investigators, many have been found to be inaccurate. It is therefore crucial to standardise spirometry, as recommended by the American Thoracic Society (ATS)/European Respiratory Society (ERS) Task Force (Box 4.2).

Performing spirometry and obtaining a reliable and reproducible result are dependent on four main criteria being met:

1. an enthusiastic, compliant subject/patient
2. a well-trained and motivated technician
3. reliable, well-maintained and correctly calibrated hardware
4. software that is appropriate to the subject/patient under investigation.

Box 4.1 Problems arising during spirometry

Technical
- Equipment itself
- Method of calculation
- Range of normal values used
- Body temperature, pressure and fully saturated (BTPS)

Practical
- Inter-spirometer variability
- Intra-spirometer variability

Accuracy (e.g. in the follow-up and monitoring of COPD)
- Smokers
- Smoking cessation
- Intervention

Box 4.2 Standardisation of spirometry, as recommended by the ATS/ERS task force

- Spirometry is a medical test that **measures** the volume or flow of air an individual inhales or exhales as a function of time
- Spirometry is an **effort-dependent** manœuvre that requires understanding, coordination and cooperation on the part of the patient/subject, who must be carefully instructed
- The **interactions** between technician and subject are crucial to obtaining adequate spirometry, as it is an effort-dependent manœuvre

SUBJECT/PATIENT

Obtaining accurate results depends on the motivation of the patient, and 'can't do' must not be confused with 'won't do'. For example, the 'can't do' reason may be important in the elderly for a variety of reasons, which may include comprehension of the instructions and coordination. A forced manœuvre may result in a worsening of existing musculoskeletal chest pain or cough, and consequently patients may 'protect themselves' from aggravating chest pain or cough by performing a suboptimal manœuvre. In children, the 'won't do' reason might be the most relevant and they will need to be appropriately coaxed in order to obtain a satisfactory result.

TECHNICIAN

Many teenage and adult subjects perform acceptable and reproducible expiratory spirometric manœuvres with a minimum of instruction and subsequent prompting. However, patients at the upper and lower end of the age range and those with severe disease in whom the results are important to subsequent management are usually more difficult cases, and accurate results may be difficult to obtain. Reliable inspiratory data are particularly difficult to collect in most patient groups.

For those reasons, a well-trained and motivated technician is crucial to providing a high-quality spirometry service. In order to achieve this, lung function tests should be performed in a quiet environment. The patient should sit upright, with the chin slightly elevated and the neck straight; this ensures that the trachea is stretched. This posture also minimises the amount of saliva that drops into the equipment.

Attention must be paid as to how the manœuvre is performed. Does the patient make sufficient effort at the beginning, when the air should be 'blasted' out? Is there a suspicion of leakage at the mouth or the mouthpiece? Does the effort end too quickly?

Visual real-time feedback on a screen during the procedure gives technicians a feeling for patient compliance and allows them to give verbal encouragement ('blow out a little harder for just a bit longer') towards the end of the manœuvre (close to residual volume (RV)) in order to achieve a reliable value for forced vital capacity (FVC, Box 4.2).

The principle of reliable spirometry is that repeated manœuvres should generate reproducible data.

Height Measurements

Predicted values of spirometry are calculated from gender, age and height. Surprisingly, standing height measurement is frequently inaccurate in practice, and careful assessment can result in values that may differ by up to 5 cm from non-standardised measurements. The main reasons include lack of proper care (e.g. removing shoes, standing completely upright) and the spinal shortening frequently present in the osteoporotic elderly patient population. A practical tip is that, in the case of unlikely results or inconsistencies in the percent predicted values between different laboratories, the possibility of height inaccuracies should be considered.

In case of spinal abnormalities, such as loss of height secondary to osteoporosis or kyphoscoliosis, arm span can be used as a surrogate way of estimating height. Arm span is the distance between the tips of the middle fingers when the arms are outstretched. This is not, however, a perfect solution, as the relationship between arm span and standing height differs slightly between ethnic groups.

Practical Recommendations for Spirometry

- Three acceptable FVC manœuvres are required.
- Acceptable repeatability is when the difference between the largest and the second largest FEV_1 and FVC is <150 mL. (For patients with an FEV_1 <1.0 L, differences between repeated measures should be <100 mL.)

If these standardisation criteria are not met in three manœuvres, additional trials should be attempted. This could involve up to, but usually no more than, eight manœuvres. Wide variability among tests is often due to incomplete inhalations. Some patients may require a brief rest period between manœuvres.

What might go wrong?

1. Poor inspiration (not filling the lungs with enough air).
2. Waiting too long at total lung capacity (TLC) before beginning the forced exhalation.
3. Not 'blasting' the air out from the onset of forced expiration.
4. Not completing the FVC manœuvre all the way to RV, and therefore producing an artificially low FVC value (Box 4.2).

What happens if the manœuvres do not fit the above criteria?

Performing the spirometry manœuvre may induce intractable cough, musculoskeletal or even cardiac chest pain, or bronchospasm, and therefore repeated attempts are unlikely to be reproducible. Children and the elderly may find completing the FVC manœuvre arduous, but may still record very reproducible FEV_1 values which, depending on the patient's age, may reflect the first 70–90% of the FVC. If the patient feels 'dizzy', the manœuvre should be stopped, since syncope could follow due to prolonged interruption of venous return to the thorax. This is more likely to occur in older subjects and those with airflow limitation. Performing a slow vital capacity (SVC) manœuvre instead of obtaining FVC may help to avoid syncope in some subjects. However, failure to meet these goals should not necessarily prevent the reporting of results, since, for some subjects, this is their best performance. Records of such manœuvres should be retained since they may contain useful information.

End-of-Test Criteria

The end of spirometry tests should come when there is no further exhalation. The technician should also terminate the test if the subject is clearly in discomfort or the volume is not continuing to increase.

HARDWARE

In a multi-centre study of 10 commonly used office spirometers that had met ATS recommendations, it was found that they scored highly on 'user-friendliness' and in general had good FEV_1 reproducibility. However, a proportional difference for FEV_1 was noted in several spirometers, which led to either an under- or an over-estimation of the results. In addition, the lack of precision of FVC and unacceptable limits of agreement between FEV_1 and FVC could result, for example, in a misclassification of chronic obstructive pulmonary disease (COPD) severity. The results implied that, for all the office spirometers tested, there was room for improvement, and cast doubt on the principle of interchangeable data between the community clinic and the lung function laboratory.

Equipment Specifications

The ATS, the European Coal and Steel Community (ECSC) and the ERS have released specification criteria, which need to be considered when using a spirometer. Unfortunately, these tend to be adhered to by the manufacturers only. The ATS equipment recommendations for diagnostic spirometry recommend a $\pm 3\%$ tolerance for vital capacity (VC) and for forced expiratory manœuvres (FVC, FEV_1).

There are two types of spirometer in common use: those that measure flow from which volume can be calculated, and those that measure volume from which flow can be calculated.

Flow-Measuring Spirometers

Air, or more specifically gas flow is measured as volume displacement per unit of time. It is measured differently depending on the type of electronic spirometer. The principle of the flow-measuring spirometers is that, in order to be accurate, the flow through these sensors must be laminar (see also pneumotachograph, Chapter 3). One disadvantage of this method is that it is sensitive to the temperature, humidity and atmospheric pressure of the surrounding air (Chapter 5). As these conditions may change, most flow-measuring spirometers must be calibrated frequently: at least daily and after each displacement. For this reason, pneumotachographs without a thermostat may not be very reliable. Classically, but not uniformly in all small commercial spirometers, the flow transducer is heated to minimise humidity in pneumotachographs and to avoid accumulation of secretions or condensation of water vapour (Figure 4.1).

Turbine Flow Meter

When a gas flows through a fixed turbine (Figure 4.2), a rotational flow is generated that drives a low-inertia vane. The rotation of the vane is converted into electrical impulses using an infrared light-emitting diode and a photodiode sensor enclosed in the turbine housing. These electrical impulses are converted into spirometric values, and the volume displacement is computed by integrating flow with respect to time, using a microprocessor in the control unit. The advantages of this system are that it is insensitive to turbulent flow, gas composition, water vapour and gas temperature if the turbine is made of carbon or Kevlar. It does not require calibration. A disadvantage of the system is its inertia, which needs to be minimised by using a very lightweight vane and applying a deflector.

Hot Wire Anemometer

This type of flow meter consists of a thin platinum wire, electrically heated to constant temperature and centrally located in a tube (Figure 4.3). As gas passes through the meter, the wire cools off, requiring extra electrical energy to maintain its temperature. The amount of electrical energy needed to reheat the wire is a proportionate measure of gas flow. Anemometers are not sensitive to the direction of the flow (inspiration, expiration), and therefore two wires are placed in series and the direction of the flow is determined from the wire that cools first.

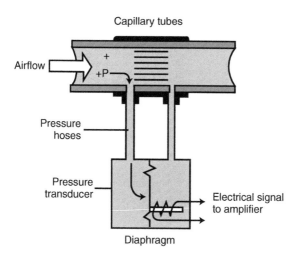

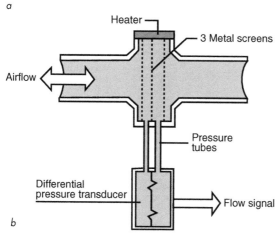

Fig. 4.1 *Structures of pneumotachographs that are commonly used in lung function laboratories.* **(a)** *Fleisch pneumotachograph;* **(b)** *Screen-type pneumotachograph. (From Cairo J, Philbeam S. Mosby's respiratory care equipment. St Louis: Mosby, 2010 with permission)*

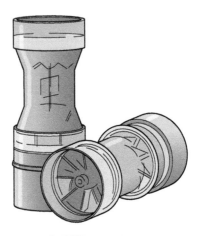

Fig. 4.2 *Structure of a turbine flow meter.*

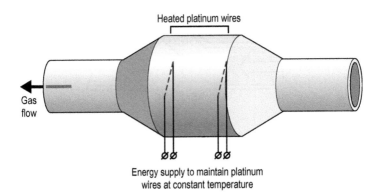

Fig. 4.3 *Structure of a hot wire anemometer.*

The output signal is linearised by a chip. The volume displacement is computed by integrating flow with respect to time. Calibration of the system must be performed frequently: at least once daily. Disadvantages of the system include sensitivity to both the composition and the temperature of the gas and undue vulnerability to damage.

Ultrasound Flow Meter

An ultrasonic sensor can be used to measure airflow. Flow is calculated from the measured gas velocity and known cross-sectional area of the gas stream (Figure 4.4). The volume is derived by integration from flow. Transducers located on either side of the cavity emit and receive sound in alternating directions. When gas flow is present in the tube, a pulse that travels against the flow (travelling upstream) is slowed down and takes longer to reach the opposite transducer. Conversely, a pulse travelling with the flow (travelling downstream) is speeded up and takes a shorter time to reach the opposite transducer. The transit time of the sound pulses is precisely measured with a digital clock. The gas flow through the spirette is calculated from the upstream and downstream transit times.

This system has no moving parts and therefore accuracy is not dependent on mechanical function; nor is it dependent on the measurement of variables such as pressure or displacement volume. Provided that the cross-sectional area of the gas stream is fixed, the only variable requiring accurate measurement is the transit time of the ultrasonic pulses between the two transmitters to receivers. These systems do not require a thermostat. Studies have shown that they are robust and that neither calibration nor linearity changes over time. One disadvantage is the expense of the main part.

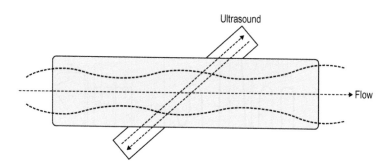

Fig. 4.4 *Structural function of a flow meter using ultrasound. Gas flow is indicated by the dotted grey lines running from left to right. In the middle section the ultrasound probe is shown sending sound waves, as indicated by the black arrows, through a defined cross-sectional area. A flow measurement can be calculated from the length of time the ultrasound pulse requires to travel through the defined space.*

Volume-Measuring Spirometers

Volume-measuring spirometers record volume over time, as flow equals volume/time. Flow can be calculated either manually or electronically. These spirometers are considered to be highly accurate as long as basic maintenance procedures are undertaken. However, they are usually significantly more bulky than the smaller portable electronic devices and therefore most often employed in lung function laboratories.

Water-Sealed Spirometer

These are the more classic type of spirometers with gas conditioning (Figure 4.5). Besides measuring spirometry, they can be used for the measurement of RV and TLC by an inert gas (such as helium) dilution technique (Chapter 6), breathing pattern and oxygen consumption. A water-sealed spirometer can be thought of as a bucket turned upside down in a water container. With exhalation, the bell is moved upward in direct proportion to the volume entering it; with inhalation, gas is withdrawn from the spirometer and the bell will move downward.

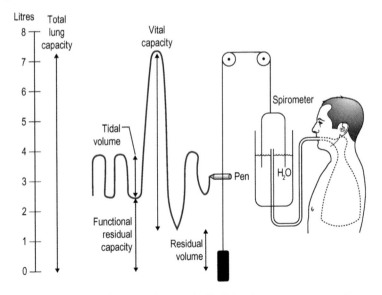

Fig. 4.5 *Structure and function of a water-sealed spirometer.*

A disadvantage of the water-sealed system is the slow response time, which makes them inappropriate for the measurement of fast volume changes. Therefore they are unsuitable for the recording of maximum inspiratory and expiratory flow–volume curves, which also excludes the accurate assessment of peak expiratory flow (PEF).

Dry Rolling Seal Spirometer

Rolling seal and wedge-bellows spirometers are equally accurate and can be used to obtain a flow–volume curve. However, they need to be adapted for measurements that entail prolonged breathing into the apparatus.

The principle behind a dry rolling seal spirometer is that of a volume-displacement type of spirometer constructed to keep mechanical resistance to a minimum (Figure 4.6). It can be altered to allow for the measurement of lung volumes, breathing pattern and oxygen consumption by adding a one-way-valve breathing circuit and CO_2 scrubber. This type of spirometer experiences problems with sticking of the rolling seal and an increased resistance in the piston-cylinder assembly.

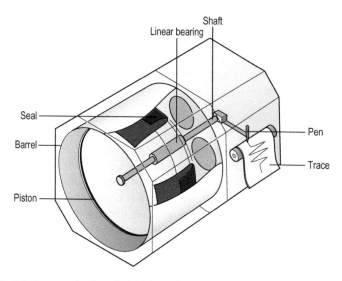

Fig. 4.6 *Structure of a dry rolling seal spirometer.*

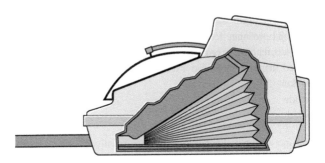

Fig. 4.7 *Structure of a wedge-bellows-type spirometer.*

Wedge-Bellows-Type Spirometer

The idea behind this kind of spirometer is that of collapsed bellows that can fold or unfold in response to changes in breathing volume (Figure 4.7). The conventional design is that of a flexible accordion-type container. One end is stationary and the other end is displaced in proportion to the inspired or exhaled volume.

Similar to the dry rolling seal spirometer, a wedge-bellows spirometer can be adapted for the measurement of lung volumes (Chapter 5) and diffusion capacity (Chapter 6) by the addition of the appropriate gas analysers and breathing circuitry.

The problems with bellows spirometry include inaccuracy from sticking of the bellows as a result of dirt or moisture. A major drawback of old bellows spirometers is that they develop air leaks in the bellows material or at the point where the bellows is mounted.

Calibration

In order to obtain accurate results from spirometry, regular calibration or monitoring is mandatory to make sure that the device has been correctly calibrated ('calibration checks'). Experience shows that, in everyday practice, calibration is frequently not carried out sufficiently; often it is not performed at all. This contrasts with the ATS/ERS guidelines, which recommend that flow-measuring spirometer calibration should be checked at least daily using a syringe of at least 3 L volume; the principle is that, if flow = volume/time, the 3 L of volume must be expelled at different velocities in order to measure a range of flows. For devices using disposable flow sensors, a new sensor from the supply used for patient tests should be tested each day.

Equally, volume-measuring spirometer calibration should be performed at least daily using a 3 L syringe. If we consider the designs of the volume spirometers (Figures 4.5–4.7), it becomes obvious that they may develop air leaks. It is therefore recommended that volume spirometers should be evaluated for leaks on a daily basis. This is checked by applying a constant positive pressure with the spirometer outlet occluded. Any observed volume loss of more than 30 mL after 1 min indicates a leak that needs to be corrected.

Biological Quality Control Check

The manufacturers' recommendation to utilise a volume syringe for calibration should be supplemented by a 'biological calibration check'. This is a periodic comparison of spirometric values obtained from a group of known healthy subjects, a method that has been shown to be relatively reliable as a way of screening for errors.

A 'biological quality control check' involves performing three technically correct spirometric manœuvres on the device, using the same healthy individual for each biological check. This is useful as a 'real-life' evaluation of the instrument's accuracy. It is reasonable to assess the overall performance of a spirometer by regularly testing a healthy individual (often a member of the laboratory personnel) every week; any variation in FEV_1 or FVC of more than 5% should result in a more exhaustive equipment evaluation.

The ATS/ERS recommendations require certain standards to be adhered to by the manufacturer but also recommend regular calibration checks. These checks should be performed on all spirometers; however, many of the electronic spirometers used outside lung function laboratories and in the community can only be checked but not calibrated. Practically, any spirometry service must undertake regular calibration checks and any significant inaccuracies must be corrected.

SOFTWARE

Predicted Values

Predicted values vary according to age, height, gender (women have smaller lungs than men) and ethnicity. This variation is better understood in a direct comparison: an elderly woman who is 1.5 m tall does not have the same lung size and compliance as a young man who is 2.0 m tall. The ideal situation is that the population to be tested has its own set of lung function prediction equations based on data acquired from that group. The range of predicted values for the elderly has only recently been extended to the age of 80 years. Testing in an immigrant-based society can be particularly problematic and predicted values should be based on local data and adjusted for ethnic-attributed variance.

Results are conventionally expressed as percent predicted, where the predicted value is derived from reference equations and the median predicted value is 100%. In practice, the normal range is between 80 and 120% predicted. As the range of 'normality' may be wider at the extremes of age (e.g. between 70 and 130% predicted), it has been suggested that the results should be expressed as z-scores (or standard deviation (SD) scores). The z-score is a mathematical combination of the % predicted and the between-subject variability into a single number that accounts for age and height-related lung function variability. However, regardless of whether the results are presented as % predicted or z-scores, an age-specific normal range should always be included in the report.

> **? Why is it important to convert absolute measures of spirometry (L and L/min) into percent predicted?**
>
> The results of spirometry have to be put into the right context if we are to understand and interpret the individual pathophysiology. Frequently, patients with a low FEV_1, as expressed in litres, may be considered as having obstructive airway disease. However, once the figures are corrected for age, height and gender by expressing the result as percent predicted, these patients may have entirely normal lung function results. This is the reason why classifications like the Global Initiative for Obstructive Lung Disease (GOLD) use percent predicted rather than absolute numbers.

In practice, a source of the reference equations used by a particular manufacturer should always be readily available. This is crucial when studying different ethnic groups, children and the elderly. New literature on the subject of predicted values is constantly emerging and software needs to be updated frequently by the manufacturers.

Influence of Weight

Height is more reliable than weight when predicting lung function, as metabolic requirements do not affect lung size (for example, obesity does not result in larger lungs). However, when following subjects over longer periods, weight changes should be considered, as the FEV_1 may decrease. The contribution of weight causing a restrictive lung defect should be taken into consideration; the mechanism is not entirely understood, however, many obese subjects do not develop a restriction at all.

Surrounding Conditions

Air and expired gases are made up of molecules and water vapour. In a gas mixture saturated with water vapour and in contact with water, as occurs in the lung, the number of water molecules in the gas phase varies with temperature and pressure. The water vapour pressure of a saturated gas is temperature-dependent. As gas volumes vary with temperature and pressure, these parameters must be recorded (see ambient temperature, pressure and saturation (ATPS)/body temperature, pressure and fully saturated (BTPS), Chapter 5).

As the water vapour pressure of a saturated gas is temperature-dependent, correction factors to convert ATPS to BTPS are used, so that, for example, 1 L of volume in ATPS at 20°C is equal to 1.102 L in BTPS conditions. Ambient temperature does have an effect on spirometric data, particularly FEV_1, and therefore it should be recorded accurately, particularly if testing is performed at temperatures above or below 23°C; testing may require continuous temperature corrections if temperature is changing rapidly. Efforts should be made to maintain the room temperature close to 23°C. Conventionally, volumes are reported at body temperature, i.e. the condition within the lungs (BTPS). The correction to BTPS adjusts for gas shrinkage due to cooling and for the condensation of water vapour, the latter being sensitive to variations in ambient barometric pressure.

The application of the conventional ATPS (ambient temperature, barometric pressure at sea level, fully saturated with water vapour) to BTPS (body temperature, barometric pressure at sea level, fully saturated with water vapour) adjustment to the volume-measuring spirometer is not entirely correct, as it is assumed that any change in gas temperature, coming from or leading to the spirometer, is accurately known and instantaneous, that the gas remains fully saturated and that the accuracy of the spirometer is not affected by temperature. Different correction factors are required for pneumotachometers and flow-measuring spirometers because the temperature of the gas as it passes through the flow sensor may vary throughout the forced manœuvre and is different for expiration and inspiration. The error will increase if the flow sensor is located further from the mouth as more cooling occurs. This is the case when a filter is placed in front of the flow sensor.

Water condensation within or on the surfaces of a flow sensor may alter its calibration. This, together with the added heat load due to the condensation of water vapour and the effect of temperature and composition on gas viscosity, increases the complexity of the applied BTPS factor.

Incorrect adjustments for BTPS are potentially a major source of inaccuracy. For example, the BTPS correction factor may be responsible for up to 10% of the measurement, depending on the environmental temperature. Changes in spirometer temperature can result in errors of up to 6% in FEV_1 and FVC if the ambient temperature is used instead of the internal spirometer temperature. Calculations used to ascertain BTPS may be inaccurate when a constant and not dynamic BTPS correction factor is used.

Infection Control

Microbial contamination of lung function equipment may result in transmission of infective diseases, although there are few confirmatory data that infections have actually been transmitted in this way. However, there is evidence to show that this is less of a problem with a test in which the patient does not inspire from the spirometer, when there is less tubing, as in most pneumotachometers, and when the pneumotachometer is heated to avoid condensation. Cross-transmission can also be a potential problem. Interestingly, some of the older water-seal spirometers were built with copper parts, and when they were exposed to water they formed copper sulphate, an effective antibacterial and antifungal agent. Nevertheless, the modern spirometer may pose the risk of presenting a source of infection, particularly for immunocompromised patients. The goal of infection control must be the prevention of the transmission of infection to the patient or to staff.

Transmission, particularly of hepatitis and human immunodeficiency virus (HIV), may be a risk due to direct contact if the patient has open sores on the oral mucosa or bleeding gums. Equally, aerosol droplets may be a source of infection in tuberculosis, and various bacterial and viral infections. These would involve mouthpieces and the immediate proximal surfaces of valves or tubing. Hand-washing discipline, especially after handling equipment and between patients, as well as the wearing of gloves, should adequately protect staff. Volume-measuring spirometers should be flushed with air between subjects and, for all spirometers, mouthpieces and any proximal tubing should be either replaced or cleaned between subjects, with more thorough cleaning on a daily basis.

Solutions to Infection Control

To avoid the transmission of infections, the recommendation is to test known infected patients at the end of the day to allow for equipment exchanges and cleaning, or to reserve equipment just for infected patients. It is also useful to have a disposable part, such as the turbine mechanism, which is changed together with the standard mouthpiece between patients. 'Antibacterial/antiviral filters' should be inserted between the disposable mouthpiece and the rest of the spirometer. The principle is that of a barrier with a certain pore size, which is small enough to prevent movement of microbes into the spirometer but not so small as to create too much flow resistance, which would influence the accuracy of the test. These filters do, however, significantly increase the resistance to flow. Although this may be statistically significant in terms of spirometric volumes, it is within the normal range of intra-individual, short-term repeatability. Calibration should be performed with the filters in place. It should be noted that these filters have not been shown to be effective against bacteria or viruses at the high flows generated at the start of a spirometric manœuvre. The use of such filters may also lead to over-reliance in terms of effective prevention of infection, resulting in a less assiduous use of existing and effective methods of infection control and hygiene such as thorough hand washing and equipment cleaning.

SUMMARY

There are multiple factors influencing the accuracy of spirometry, depending on the equipment used, staff experience, patient motivation, software and reference equations applied. Environmental factors, such as ATPS and BTPS, have to be considered (Box 4.3). It is crucial that measures of infection control are applied to avoid transmission of airborne or other diseases to the patient being tested or to staff.

Box 4.3 Schematic summary of factors influencing accuracy of spirometry

- Range of inaccuracy greater than ATS/ERS recommendations
- Correction to BTPS: errors up to 10%
- Slow response time: errors up to 15%
- Need for improved methods of calibration

CHAPTER 5

Lung Volume Measurements

KEY POINTS

- Measurement of lung volumes provides important additional clinical information in diagnosis and management over and above that provided by spirometry. Lung volume measurements are essential in the diagnosis of hyperinflation and restriction, and to understanding the pathophysiological principles behind them.
- Lung volume measurements are most commonly performed using body plethysmography or helium dilution method.
- In obstructive disease, lung volume can identify relative and absolute levels of hyperinflation. In restrictive disease, a reduced total lung capacity determines the level of restriction. Measurement of lung volumes will elucidate suspicions of a combined obstructive and restrictive ventilatory defect derived from spirometric data.
- There are limitations to the accurate measurement of lung volume if the technical aspects are not correctly addressed. These include limitation of the gas dilution technique in severe airway obstruction, potential sources of inaccuracy in body plethysmography measurements, and variability in reference equations.

Why do we need to measure lung volumes?

Lung volumes may be reduced in restrictive disease and increased in obstructive disease; these changes may not be obvious from simple spirometry.

BACKGROUND – WHAT WE CANNOT MEASURE WITH SPIROMETRY

Spirometry requires full inhalation to total lung capacity (TLC); the total exhaled volume measured at the mouth is the vital capacity (VC), which therefore does not include the measure of residual volume (RV). RV cannot be measured directly by analysing volume at the mouth but nevertheless accounts for approximately 20% of TLC in normal subjects.

The difference between the forced (FVC) and slow vital capacity (SVC) manœuvres is usually small. However, in patients with significant chronic airway obstruction, for example, the FVC may be significantly less than the SVC, as a result of air being trapped in the lung secondary to airway collapse. The finding of a significant difference between FVC and SVC should lead to additional measurements, particularly the determination of lung volumes (Figure 3.1).

INTRODUCTION

The measurement of lung volumes offers more specific information and diagnostic accuracy than spirometry alone, but requires expensive and bulky equipment. There are two established standard methods used for lung volume measurements: the helium dilution method and the body plethysmography. The nitrogen washout method and imaging techniques (X-ray, computed tomography, magnetic resonance imaging, optometrical plethysmography) offer alternative methods, but are less frequently used as standard measurements in lung function laboratories.

The helium dilution technique and the body plethysmography method evolved around the mid-20th century. In addition to standard dynamic and static volume measurements, as derived from spirometry, such measurement of lung volumes allows the non-invasive determination of RV, functional residual capacity (FRC) or intrathoracic gas volume (ITGV), TLC and airway resistance.

Gas Dilution Method

Along with body plethysmography, the gas dilution method is the most commonly used method of determining lung volumes. It is usually based on the use of a tracer gas (such as helium) that is inhaled in a defined concentration until equilibration is reached, and then measured again in expiration. The degree of dilution allows calculation of the volume of gas that has been interacting with the inhaled gas in

Table 5.1 Different lung volume measurements and their meaning, with units

Parameter	Definition	Abbreviation(s)	Unit
Airway resistance	Pressure gradient between mouth and alveolar space	R_{aw}	$kPa* s* L^{-1}$
Specific airway resistance	This is not an ohm resistance in the physical sense; product of specific resistance and ITGV	sR_{aw}	$kPa* s$
Airway conductance	Reciprocal of airway resistance; the instantaneous rate of gas flow per unit of pressure difference between the mouth, nose or other airway opening and the alveoli	G_{aw}	$kPa^{-1}* s^{-1}* L$
Specific airway conductance	Conductance corrected for lung volume	sG_{aw}	$kPa^{-1}* s^{-1}$
Intrathoracic gas volume	Volume inside the chest at end-expiration, measured by body plethysmography; also contains trapped intrathoracic and intra-abdominal air not participating in ventilation	ITGV, TGV, IGV	L
Functional residual capacity	Comparable to ITGV; measured by helium dilution technique; contains only ventilated ITGV	FRC	L
Total lung capacity	The entire lung volume at full inflation	TLC	L
Residual volume	Remaining volume at maximal expiration	RV	L

the lung. The method requires the tracer gas to be inert and insoluble, so that minimal amounts of it diffuse into the lung parenchyma and the blood. The gas dilution method facilitates determination of FRC (Table 5.1). An alternative way to determine lung volumes uses nitrogen in an elimination technique.

Body Plethysmography Principle

The underlying principle of body plethysmography is that the product of pressure (P) and volume (V) in a closed isothermic system of gas is constant

($P \times V = $ constant; Boyle's law). Body box measurements employ either the constant volume or the constant pressure principle. In constant volume measurements, the volume of the body plethysmograph box is kept constant and pressure changes during resting breathing inside the box are recorded. Similarly, with constant pressure registration, the pressures are kept constant while the change of volume with tidal breathing is recorded. Constant pressure body plethysmograph boxes do not have to consider body volume and are less sensitive to air leaks (Table 5.1).

> ### ❓ How should we approach lung volume measurements in practice?
>
> The measurement of lung volumes employs a stepwise approach to assess ventilation, symptoms and diseases of the respiratory system. Usually, the first investigation is spirometry. However, additional measurements of lung volumes and resistance offer more specific information and diagnostic accuracy (Figure 3.1).

INDICATIONS FOR LUNG VOLUME MEASUREMENTS

The body plethysmography and helium dilution methods usually yield similar results for FEV_1, SVC and FVC because, following measurement of FRC or ITGV and airway resistance, the same manœuvres are performed to derive TLC or RV. However, lung volume measurements allow the following:

1. Diagnosis of hyperinflation
2. Quantification of restrictive lung disease
3. Further assessment of symptoms (breathlessness, cough, sputum).
4. Quantification of obstructive airway and lung disease
5. Diagnosis of airway stenosis
6. Follow-up of diagnosed respiratory disease
7. Airway obstruction reversibility and provocation tests
8. Assessment of indications for therapy and treatment efficacy
9. Objective measurement of adverse events
10. Assessment of procedural risk
11. Occupational follow-up for professions at risk
12. Assessment of health status for social services or benefits.

METHODS AND MEASUREMENTS

Gas Dilution Techniques

Equation 5.1

Gas Dilution Principle

$$V_1 \, C_1 = V_2 \, C_2$$

If the volume of the circuit system (V_1) and the concentration of the tracer gas in it (C_1) are known, and the concentration of the gas in expiration (C_2) can be measured, then the volume of the circuit plus lung volume (V_2) can be derived from the equation above. The lung volume is calculated as $V_2 - V_1$.

For the gas dilution method, the patient starts to breathe the test gas (usually a mixture of 10% helium, 25–30% oxygen (O_2) and balanced nitrogen is used to fill the circuit system) at the end of a normal tidal expiration and is then instructed to breathe with regular tidal breaths (Figure 3.1; Equation 5.1). The O_2 flow is adjusted to compensate for O_2 consumption, as significant errors in the calculation of FRC levels can result if it is not adequately accounted for. The helium concentration is noted periodically and helium equilibration is considered to be complete when the change in helium concentration becomes minimal over a period of approximately 30 seconds. Equilibration will take longer in very obstructed patients, and may take as long as 10 minutes in patients with severe gas-exchange abnormalities. In normal subjects there is relatively good agreement between measurements using the helium dilution method and body plethysmography. In chronic obstructive pulmonary disease (COPD), particularly if this is moderate to severe, the differences between FRC and ITGV (Table 5.1) increase significantly as the inert gas fails to reach all lung areas (this can be more than 600 mL) and therefore may significantly underestimate lung volumes. This effect is particularly marked in bullous emphysema, when the bullae have little connection to the airway. However, if enough time is allowed for gas equilibration, the FRC_{He}–$ITGV_{Body}$ difference can be minimised in most obstructed patients.

The helium (or nitrogen) dilution methods can be used either in the form of a single-breath method or as a multiple-breath equilibrium technique. The single-breath method entails inhaling to full inflation, i.e. to TLC, followed by a 10 s breath-hold and then rapid exhalation. With helium, a tracer gas is inhaled in an equilibration method; with nitrogen, 100% oxygen is inhaled and the nitrogen washout concentration is measured to calculate lung volumes. Alveolar volume (V_A), which is the lung volume that can be calculated simultaneously with the measurement of the transfer factor (TLCO), is about 5% less than the TLC measured by the multi-breath helium technique in normal subjects. However, this technique is considerably less accurate in the presence of significant airway obstruction. Lung volume measurements derived from the single-breath method are commonly abbreviated and indexed as V_A (TLCO–V_A).

Body Plethysmography Technique

The principle of body plethysmography is based on Boyle's law which states that, at constant temperature in a defined space, the changes in pressure (P) and volume (V) are inversely correlated (Equation 5.2). This means that the product of pressure and volume remains constant, and with pressures and volumes measured, lung volume can be derived by the changes recorded.

E$_Q$ Equation 5.2

Modified Boyle's Law

$$P_1 V_1 = P_2 V_2$$

P_1 = alveolar pressure at time 1, P_2 = alveolar pressure at time 2, V_1 = lung volume at time 1, V_2 = lung volume at time 2.

The product of pressure and volume is constant. When panting against airway occlusion (shutter on the mouthpiece), pressure changes and volume changes in lung volume (expansion/compression) can be recorded, and lung volume (ITGV) can be calculated.

Body Temperature and Pressure, Fully Saturated (BTPS)

Air and expired gas are made up of gas molecules and water vapour. In a gas mixture saturated with water vapour and in contact with water (such as occurs in the lung), the number of water molecules in the gas phase varies with temperature and pressure. The water vapour pressure of a saturated gas is temperature-dependent. As gas volumes vary with temperature and pressure, these parameters must be recorded.

What is BTPS?
Lung volumes and flows are standardized to body temperature, barometric pressure at sea level, saturated with water vapour.

What is ATPS?
Lung volumes and flows are standardized to ambient temperature, barometric pressure at sea level, saturated with water vapour.

In order to measure lung volumes using a body plethysmograph, the patient first needs to be seated within the box itself (Figure 5.1). The patient then breathes through a mouthpiece into a pneumotachograph, while wearing a nose clip.

The patient will be asked to breathe in and out quietly. Firstly, specific airway resistance (sR_{aw}) is measured; this is an assessment of airway resistance made during tidal breathing. Once the patient reaches the end-expiratory baseline at rest, the shutter is closed abruptly and the patient is asked to continue to breathe in and out slowly against the resistance created. This is followed by the manœuvre to determine ITGV (Figure 5.2). Further, dynamic and static lung volumes will be derived from a spirometry manœuvre in the body box.

The underlying assumption of the technique is that the pressure–volume changes in the body are isothermal, and that any heat generated by compression is instantaneously lost to the surrounding tissue. The changes in pressure and volume within the plethysmograph are assumed to be adiabatic (which means that there is insufficient time for heat exchange to occur between the air within the plethysmograph and either the walls or the subject during the rarefaction and compression manœuvre). Panting frequencies are therefore kept very slow (in the order of 0.5–1 Hz) for reasons of measurement accuracy.

Pressure–Flow Diagram

While the patient is breathing at rest, pressure changes in the body plethysmograph are registered. A diagram is plotted on which the pressure is visualised on the x-axis. In parallel, flow is registered via the mouthpiece and a pneumotachograph on the y-axis, creating a pressure–flow diagram (Figure 5.3). This plot provides useful information, and the specific airway resistance can be calculated (Figure 5.4).

The product of pressure and volume is constant, according to Boyle's law (Equation 5.2). Thus, for measurement of the ITGV, it is necessary to assume that

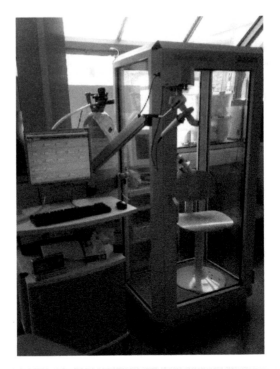

Fig. 5.1 *Modern body plethysmograph (constant-volume box) with computer terminal.*

pressure changes in the body box are negative, proportional to those in the alveolar space. For this particular measurement, as mentioned earlier, the shutter will be closed in end-expiration so that the patient is breathing in and out against an occluded airway (slow panting). This time, pressure changes inside the body plethysmograph will be plotted on the x-axis, and pressure changes on the mouthpiece on the y-axis (Figure 5.4). ITGV can now be derived from the tangent of the angle between the curve and the x-axis (Figure 5.5).

DIFFERENT LUNG VOLUME PARAMETERS

The most important parameters derived from body plethysmography or helium dilution method are summarised in Table 5.1.

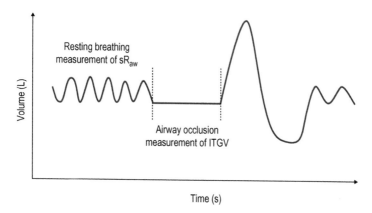

Fig. 5.2 Breathing manœuvre to measure specific airway resistance (sR$_{aw}$) and intrathoracic gas volume (ITGV) with a body plethysmograph. Firstly, tidal breathing is recorded, followed by an airway occlusion with a shutter. Once the shutter reopens, the patient takes a deep breath to TLC and blows out to RV. The absolute level of lung volume (ITGV) must be related to fixed lung volumes such as TLC and RV.

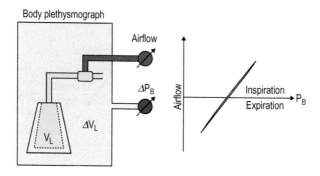

Fig. 5.3 Schematic picture of the measurement of a Pressure–Flow curve. The x-axis registers pressure changes (ΔP) in the body box; the y-axis plots the airflow. ΔP_B = change of pressure in the body plethysmograph, ΔV_L = change of lung volume.

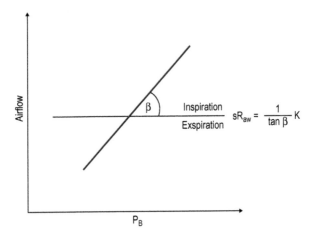

Fig. 5.4 Deriving the specific airway resistance (sR_aw) from the pressure–flow curve. K = calibration factor.

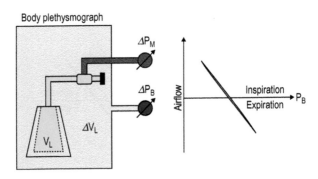

Fig. 5.5 Schematic picture of the measurement of the pressure curve. The x-axis registers pressure changes (ΔP) in the body box; the y-axis plots the changes in mouth pressure. ΔP_B = change of pressure in the body plethysmograph, ΔP_M = change of mouth pressure.

Airway Resistance (R_{aw})

The airway resistance (R_{aw}) is defined as pressure loss in the respiratory system per unit of flow (Equation 5.3). It is a marker of the width of the central airways (approximately first to eighth airway generation). The narrower the airway, the larger the airway resistance. Increased airway resistance at rest is frequently observed with obstructive ventilatory disease, but can also be found with extra-thoracic stenosis, e.g. laryngeal carcinoma, or vocal cord dysfunction. Airway resistance can also be increased in restrictive ventilatory disorders as a result of tidal breathing at a lower lung volume (Figure 2.11), and of the associated narrower airways.

 Equation 5.3

Airway Resistance (R_{aw})

$$R_{aw} = \frac{\tan \alpha}{\tan \beta} K$$

Specific Airway Resistance (sR_{aw})

The specific airway resistance has the unit kPa *s, and as such is not a resistance according to Ohm's law. The specific airway resistance, in contrast to R_{aw}, can be derived even if it seems to be impossible to record a proper occlusion curve, e.g. due to lack of motivation. It is therefore controlled for confounding factors due to shift of lung volumes at tidal breathing.

Resistance Measured by Oscillation (R_{osc})

Airway resistance can be measured using oscillation of the air by high frequencies. The oscillating air in the airways allows derivation of the unknown resistance (R_{osc}) by considering changes in pressure and airflow compared to a known resistance. The interpretation of the results is similar to the bronchial airway resistance, as measured by body plethysmography (R_{aw}).

Different resistances of the airways may also be measured using multi-frequency oscillometry, which analyses the reactance to different sound signals of multiple frequencies (5–35 Hz). This method allows the recording of impedance (Z) and characterisation of the airways with a complex spectrum of impedance over a range of frequencies. Impedance includes the real airflow resistance (R) and an imaginary resistance derived from the interference of capacitive and inertive energy storage (Reactance X). Resistance causes loss of energy, but negative reactance leads to capacitive (Capacitance C) and positive reactance to inertive (Inertance I) energy storage. Additionally, it is recorded where the reactance is '0', this frequency is called resonance frequency (F_{res}).

The method is still being developed, but it may have value in early recognition of airway disease due to high sensitivity. It is also easy to use in children, as it requires less volitional effort than other lung function tests.

Intrathoracic Gas Volume (ITGV) and Functional Residual Capacity (FRC)

ITGV and FRC are the volumes that remain in the lung at end-expiration and that equal balanced elastic forces. While ITGV is measured using body plethysmography (Figures 5.5 and 5.6), FRC is derived using the helium dilution method. ITGV and FRC are somewhat comparable, but ITGV includes intrathoracic gas that is not participating in ventilation, resulting in a higher ITGV than FRC in older

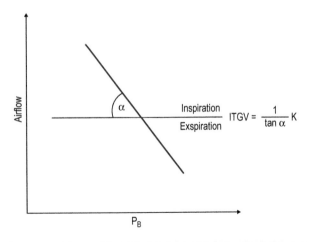

Fig. 5.6 *Derivation of the intrathoracic gas volume (ITGV) using the occlusion pressure method. K = calibration factor.*

or obstructive patients. It is therefore found to be higher in patients with hyper-inflation due to COPD. Restrictive ventilatory disorders tend to have lower ITGV or FRC volumes.

Total Lung Capacity

TLC is the lung volume at maximal inspiration. It can be greatly increased in ob-structive ventilatory disease due to hyperinflation. In order to classify a restrictive lung disease, TLC must be reduced.

Residual Volume

This is the volume that remains in the lung with maximal expiration. It can be in-creased in obstructive lung disease, and the ratio between residual volume and total lung capacity (RV/TLC) is increased in hyperinflation. In restrictive disease, the residual volume can be decreased.

 What do the results of these measurements tell me?

For most of the lung volumes and spirometry results, there are comparative tables that consider age, gender and height when determining predicted normal parameters. In addition, a set of predicted normal values should be available for each ethnic population, if possible. However, there may be significant variability, even in the test results expressed as percent predicted, in the same patient between different lung function laboratories. It is important to understand that changes in lung volumes over time, using the same equipment in the same laboratory, may offer more information than different measurements from different laboratories.

SPECIFIC RESULTS IN VENTILATORY DISEASES

Ventilatory diseases are differentiated into obstructive, restrictive and mixed pat-terns. An obstructive disease is characterised by a diminished FEV_1/FVC ratio and an increased airway resistance (R_{aw}). In contrast, a restrictive ventilatory dis-ease is defined by a reduction in total lung capacity (TLC). A decrease in vital capacity may suggest restriction if only spirometry is available, but in this case the FEV_1/FVC ratio is usually normal to exclude an obstruction and the Flow–Volume curve must be normal in appearance (Figure 5.7). However, a reduced FVC could also be a result of an increased RV, resulting in a normal or close to

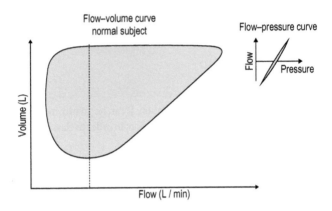

Fig. 5.7 Normal Flow–Volume and Flow–Pressure curves.

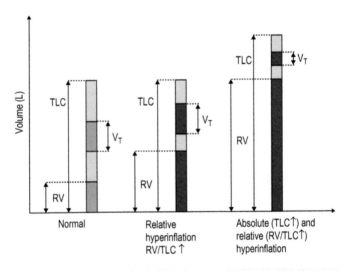

Fig. 5.8 Schematic changes in lung volume between normal subjects and patients with relative hyperinflation (normal TLC and elevated RV/TLC ratio) and absolute hyperinflation (TLC ↑). RV = residual volume, TLC = total lung capacity, ↑ = increased, V_T = tidal volume.

normal FEV_1/FVC ratio despite obstructive pathology (Figure 5.8). It is therefore necessary to have a normal FEV_1/FVC ratio and a normal appearance of the Flow–Volume loop to exclude obstruction. A mixed disease has both characteristics, i.e. a decreased TLC and a diminished FEV_1/FVC ratio.

Obstructive Disease

An airway obstruction is caused by an increase in airway resistance when intra-thoracic or extrathoracic narrowing of the airway leads to a diminished FEV_1 and decreased FEV_1/FVC ratio, often combined with hyperinflation (Figure 5.8). The most common causes of airway obstruction are summarised in the following list:

1. Bronchial asthma
2. Chronic obstructive bronchitis and/or bronchiectasis
3. Lung emphysema
4. Bronchiolitis
5. Laryngeal disease (e.g. tumour, oedema, vocal cord dysfunction)
6. Tracheal compression or tumour, tracheomalacia
7. Central bronchial tumour.

A good indicator of airway obstruction is the Flow–Volume curve. A 'kinking' or scalloping of the expiratory part of this curve is caused by reduced airflow velocity (Figure 5.9).

Flow–Volume curves in patients with obstructive emphysema, asthma and fixed airway stenosis are shown in Figures 5.10 and 5.11.

An example of how the Flow–Volume curve may change following a reversibility test is shown in Figure 5.12.

The measurement of airway resistance may allow assessment of patients who are unable to perform good spirometric manœuvres.

? Does a reduced FEV_1 mean that the patient has airway obstruction?

An isolated low FEV_1 does not diagnose airway obstruction. Only when it is related to the vital capacity (FEV_1/FVC ratio) that diagnosis can be made. In restrictive disease the FEV_1 can also be low, but in relation to the existing FVC it is normal. It is also important to keep in mind that some patients may have concurrent restrictive and obstructive disease.

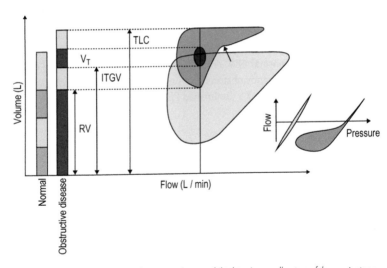

Fig. 5.9 Obstructive airway disease with typical 'kinking' or scalloping of the expiratory flow (arrow) in the Flow–Volume curve and a characteristic change of the Flow–Pressure curve in the shape of a golf club (right). Normal curves are coloured blue; obstructive curves are pink. ITGV = intrathoracic gas volume, RV = residual volume, TLC = total lung capacity, V_T = tidal volume.

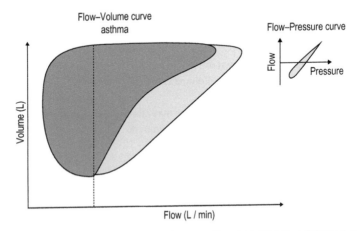

Fig. 5.10 Typical example of Flow–Volume and Flow–Pressure curves in asthma. There is slightly diminished peak flow (PEF) and more reduced FEF_{75}, FEF_{50} and FEF_{25} as markers of small airway obstruction. Normal curves are coloured blue, obstructive pink.

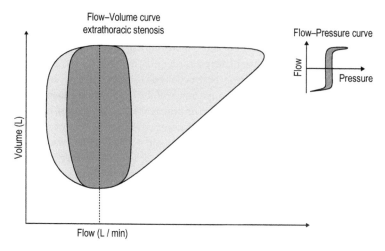

Fig. 5.11 Example for a Flow-Volume curve with fixed airway stenosis.

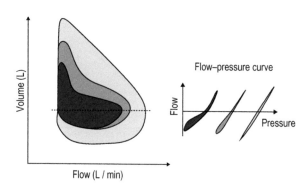

Fig. 5.12 Flow–Volume and Flow–Pressure curves for obstructive ventilatory disease prior to (red) and following (pink) bronchodilatation with beta$_2$-agonists. Peak flow and expiratory airflow are higher following broncholysis, indicating partial reversibility. Normal predicted lung function is displayed in blue.

Restrictive Disease

Restriction is defined by reduced TLC (Figure 5.13). In cases where TLC cannot be measured, a restrictive ventilatory disorder may be consistent with a reduction in vital capacity (VC). Airway obstruction has to be excluded, which means that the FEV_1/FVC ratio and the appearance of the Flow–Volume loop should be normal. This is necessary because an obstructive ventilatory disease may lead to hyperinflation with increased RV and lower vital capacity (Figures 5.8 and 5.9). There are multiple reasons for developing a restriction, which may primarily be distinguished by their pulmonary or extrapulmonary aetiology. Pulmonary causes of restriction (e.g. lung fibrosis) may be identified by a relatively high PEF, which is attributed to changed compliance of the lung, a measure of the elasticity, with fast retraction following full inflation (Figure 5.14; Chapter 2). Measurement of diffusion can provide useful information for the differential diagnosis (Chapter 6). Causes of restrictive defects on lung function tests may be summarised as shown in Box 5.1.

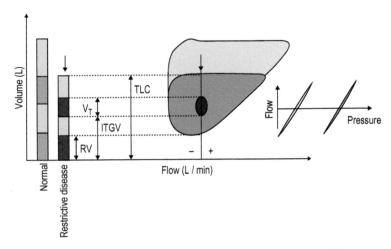

Fig. 5.13 *Representative example for a restrictive disease with decreased TLC (arrows) and vital capacity. ITGV = intrathoracic gas volume, RV = residual volume, TLC = total lung capacity, V_T = tidal volume.*

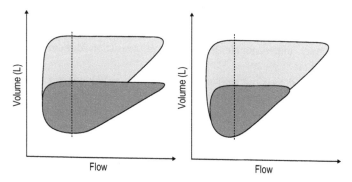

Fig. 5.14 *Normal Flow–Volume curve (blue) and with restriction (pink). The left panel shows an example of displacement of the curve with pulmonary restriction, the right panel with extrapulmonary restriction.*

Box 5.1 Causes of restrictive defects on lung function tests

Pulmonary/Diseases of the Lung
- Local diseases (e.g. pulmonary fibrosis, tumours, pneumonia, atelectasis)
- Generalised organ involvement (e.g. congestion, rheumatic disorders)

Extrapulmonary/Diseases of the Pleura
- Effusion
  - Exudate
  - Transudate
  - Empyema
- Pneumothorax
- Non-specific thickening of the pleura (e.g. scar tissue, malignancy)

Extrapulmonary/Diseases of the Chest Wall and Respiratory Muscle Pump
- Musculoskeletal (e.g. neural, neuromuscular junction or muscular disorders)
  - Congenital (e.g. neuromuscular disease, scoliosis)
  - Acquired (e.g. myasthenia gravis, Lambert–Eaton syndrome, diaphragmatic paralysis, amyotrophic lateral sclerosis)
- Trauma

The degree of restrictive ventilatory defect is reported according to the percent change from predicted values. A combination of obstruction and restriction may underestimate the degree of restriction due to secondary hyperinflation.

Restrictive defects can be diagnosed when TLC is reduced to less than the 5th percentile of the predicted normal population (American Thoracic Society (ATS)/European Respiratory Society (ERS), 1995 or European Coal and Steel Community (ECSC), 1993). A reduced vital capacity alone does not prove restriction, but it may be suggestive when the FEV_1/FVC ratio is normal or increased. A low TLC from a single-breath test can severely underestimate lung volumes and should not be seen as evidence of restriction.

 Why is it important to look at the recorded traces?

Ventilatory diseases are often characterised by typical deviations and identified by disease-specific patterns. It is therefore important not only to look at single numbers (e.g. FEV_1) but to look at them in the context of the overall picture. The Flow–Volume curve and standard printouts from the lung function laboratory allow such identification and, in a single view, may point the way towards a diagnosis.

Combined or Mixed Ventilatory Defects

In a mixed ventilatory pattern, both TLC and FEV_1/FVC ratio may be reduced (Figure 5.15); this cannot be accurately diagnosed by spirometry alone.

Common causes for this are:

1. Cystic fibrosis
2. Bronchiectasis
3. COPD plus loss of functional lung tissue
4. Post-tuberculosis
5. Silicosis and asbestosis
6. Sarcoidosis.

A summary of how to interpret lung function test results is given in Figure 5.16. The lower limit of normal is defined as below the 5th percentile in a normal healthy population. Most lung function laboratories use either the

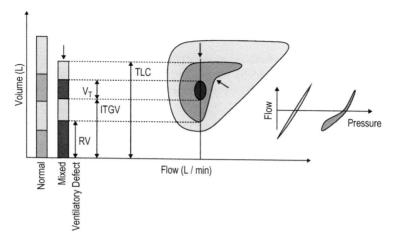

Fig. 5.15 Flow–Volume curve and Flow–Pressure curve in a mixed ventilatory defect. Arrows indicate reduced TLC and obstructive airflow in expiration. ITGV = intrathoracic gas volume, RV = residual volume, TLC = total lung capacity, V_T = tidal volume.

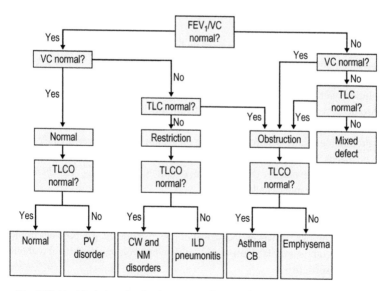

Fig. 5.16 Modified algorithm for the interpretation of lung function test results. CB = chronic bronchitis, CW and NM disorders = chest wall and neuromuscular disorders, ILD = interstitial lung disease, PV disorders = pulmonary vascular disorders, TLCO = transfer factor.
(Adapted from 'ATS/ERS Standardisation of lung function testing – interpretative strategies for lung function testing'. Eur Respir J 2005;26:948–968 with permission)

ATS/ERS workshop references or the equations from the ECSC. Recently, reference values for the elderly were published (Garcia-Rio et al.). However, individual ethnic communities are encouraged to compile their own predicted values tables.

PITFALLS IN LUNG VOLUME MEASUREMENTS

Despite the fact that measurement of lung volumes is important in the diagnosis, management and prognosis of the majority of respiratory disorders, the available techniques demand considerable skill and expertise.

The gas dilution techniques require gas supplies, appropriate analysers and a long period of rebreathing, which can be demanding for patients. The most important limitation is the fact that tracer gases (usually helium and nitrogen) may not reach the more poorly ventilated regions of the lung in patients with more severe chronic airway obstruction, and this results in underestimation of lung volumes. Commercial systems frequently limit equilibration time to no more than 4 to 5 minutes.

Body plethysmography is the most widely used method and is the accepted 'gold standard' for lung volume measurements. However, measuring TLC by this technique tends to overestimate lung volumes compared to the helium dilution method, even in normal subjects, and the effect is exaggerated in chronic airway obstruction. It is a relatively quick procedure if performed by a proficient, well-trained technician. However, achievement of reliable and reproducible results is more demanding on the operator and even on the patient (who needs to cooperate more fully) than for the gas dilution techniques. Equipment is expensive and is more reliant on electronics, which makes troubleshooting more challenging.

Imaging techniques are not currently in routine clinical use, as they are poorly validated and may (depending on the technique) expose the patient to a significant radiation risk. However, the arrival of new technology, e.g. opto-electronic plethysmography, may facilitate more accurate lung volume assessment without radiation exposure.

SUMMARY

The addition of lung volume measurements to the static and dynamic parameters derived from spirometry, along with the measurement of airway resistance, can provide valuable information. Body plethysmography facilitates measurement of intrathoracic gas volume, total lung capacity and airway resistance, whilst the helium dilution method determines functional residual capacity and total lung capacity. Lung volume measurements are necessary to diagnose obstructive or restrictive disease, assess respiratory symptoms, follow disease progression, document the effect of therapeutic interventions, and identify peri-procedural risks.

CHAPTER 6

Diffusion, Gas Exchange and Blood Gas Measurements

KEY POINTS: DIFFUSION AND GAS EXCHANGE

- The usual indicator gas for diffusion measurement is carbon monoxide (CO).
- CO binds more than 200 times better to haemoglobin than oxygen (O_2); full saturation is achieved with a partial pressure of <1 mmHg of CO.
- TLCO (DLCO) is derived from the quotient of CO take-up (V_{CO}) and the alveolo-capillary CO partial pressure difference. Thus, TLCO (DLCO) = $V_{CO}/paCO$ (mL/min/mmHg).
- Single-breath method: calculation of V_{CO} after full inhalation of an air mixture containing 0.2% CO followed by an apnoea of 10 s. For an accurate measurement, the alveolar volume (V_A) has to be known.
- Steady-state method: the patient breathes an air mixture with 0.1% CO for 3–5 min, until a steady state is reached. V_{CO} is derived from the end-expiratory exhaled air mix.

KEY POINTS: BLOOD GASES

- Blood gases can be analysed in an arterial blood sample, which is usually taken from the radial artery, or from an arterialised blood sample taken from the earlobe.
- Arterial blood gas analysis yields partial pressure of oxygen (paO_2), partial pressure of carbon dioxide ($paCO_2$) and H^+ ions. Other parameters (bicarbonate, base excess) are calculated and derived from these measurements.
- The blood gas analysis can identify compensated or uncompensated acidotic or alkalotic conditions. It can help to determine the respiratory or metabolic origin of an alkalosis or acidosis.

DIFFUSION AND GAS EXCHANGE: INTRODUCTION

The single-breath CO transfer factor measurement diagnoses impaired gas exchange. The transfer factor (TLCO) for carbon monoxide, sometimes termed the diffusing capacity (DLCO), is defined as the amount of CO gas that diffuses through the alveolo-capillary membrane in a defined time and with known partial pressures of gas tension. In addition, the transfer coefficient K_L (Krogh index) can be derived as the CO gas that is taken up per time relative to the ventilated volume, V_A (TLCO/V_A). An isolated reduction of the TLCO (DLCO) is found in the presence of a reduced area available for diffusion (gas exchange disorder), while an additional reduction of the Krogh index indicates a diffusion disorder.

 What do measurements of gas exchange add to lung volume measures and spirometry?

Spirometry (see Chapter 3) and lung volume measurements (see Chapter 5) are markers of lung and airway size, but measuring the gas exchange at the air–blood barrier can help to identify disturbed oxygen uptake capacity, e.g. in interstitial lung or vascular diseases.

BACKGROUND

Gas exchange is the primary function of the respiratory system. The TLCO (DLCO) of the lung is defined as gas transfer capacity of carbon monoxide (CO), and the CO partial pressure difference between the alveolar space and pulmonary capillaries quantifies the amount of gas diffusing through the alveolo-capillary membrane. The most widely used technique is the so-called 'single-breath method'. The advantage of this method is that it is easy and quickly available, but it depends on patient motivation and is therefore not always reliable. The single-breath CO transfer factor method quantifies gas exchange disorders that most commonly affect oxygen uptake and not necessarily CO_2 elimination, because CO_2 has an approximately 20 times higher diffusion capacity than O_2.

There are multiple reasons why the transfer factor may be low. In addition to pathological changes in the diffusion area and membrane, distribution and perfusion inequalities or anaemia may contribute to a low transfer factor. Low levels of CO are inhaled during the measurement, as the mean venous partial pressure of CO can usually be assumed to be '0' (notable exceptions are heavy smokers and patients with CO intoxication). In all other cases, it is sufficient to measure only alveolar partial pressure of CO. Modern blood gas analysers facilitate the measurement of CO haemoglobin, which can be used to correct for transfer factor measurements independent of CO content in the blood. In addition to the transfer factor measurement, helium is mixed into the inhaled gas mixture, which allows calculation of the ventilated volume during the same manœuvre.

The added helium also facilitates an evaluation of total lung capacity (TLC), and subtraction of vital capacity yields residual volume (RV). In contrast to body plethysmography, only ventilated lung areas are measured with this method. In certain conditions, e.g. emphysema with significant trapped air, the TLC, as measured by the body plethysmograph, may be larger than obtained by the helium dilution technique ($TLC_B > TLC_{He}$, Chapter 5). This difference tends to be even more pronounced when measured by a single breath, as opposed to a multi-breath technique.

MEASUREMENT

There are two different manœuvres to measure the diffusion capacity of the lungs: the single-breath (SB) method and the steady-state (SS) method. For the single-breath measurement, the patient is seated, wearing a nose clip and breathing in a relaxed way via a mouthpiece. The patient is asked to exhale to RV, followed by a maximal inspiratory manœuvre (IVC) up to TLC. This manœuvre should be completed within 3 s and followed by breath-holding lasting 8–10 s. During this manœuvre, the patient inhales a CO-helium gas mixture. Immediately after breath-holding, the patient performs a forced vital capacity manœuvre and the expired air is analysed for the remaining gas concentrations, following deduction of the dead space. The minimal amount of air required for an accurate measurement should be between 0.6 and 0.9 L and the manœuvre should not last longer than 3 s (Figure 6.1).

The steady-state method involves a similar set-up, but the patient is continuously breathing an air mixture with low levels of CO as a marker gas for 3–5 min, or until a steady state is reached and V_{CO} is measured in the exhaled gases. The most important parameters derived from the CO transfer factor measurements are listed in Table 6.1.

107

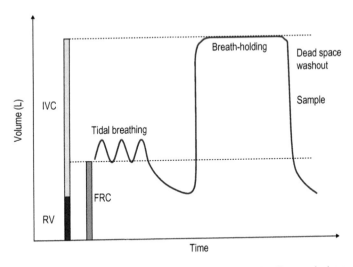

Fig. 6.1 Breathing manœuvre for measurement of TLCO (DLCO). The sample that is analysed for the inhaled concentration of CO is collected during expiration following an appropriate dead-space washout. FRC = functional residual capacity, IVC = inspiratory vital capacity, RV = residual volume.

Table 6.1 Parameters derived from the diffusion capacity measurement		
Parameter	**Definition**	**Unit**
TLCO (DLCO)	Carbon monoxide transfer factor; gas amount that is exchanged between the alveolar space and erythrocytes; marker for oxygen uptake	mmol/min/kPa (or mmol/min/ mmHg)
V_A	Ventilated volume	L
TLCO/V_A (DLCO/V_A) or KCO	Krogh index, rate-constant amount of gas exchanged between the alveolar space and erythrocytes relative to the ventilated volume	mmol/min/ kPa/L
TLC_{He}	Total lung capacity, as measured by the helium dilution method	L
HbCO	Carboxyhaemoglobin, percent of HB with CO (increased with smoking)	%

PREDICTED VALUES

According to the recommendations of the American Thoracic Society (ATS), each lung function laboratory should measure a sufficient number of healthy subjects and compare the results with the different reference equations to determine the best prediction equation for that local reference population. For this purpose, a minimum number of 15 healthy male and 15 healthy female subjects should be included. However, one of the most commonly used published reference equations has been described by Cotes et al. (European Coal and Steel Community, 1993).

INTERPRETATION OF THE MEASUREMENT

For the interpretation of the test results it is necessary to consider the TLCO (DLCO) for CO and the transfer coefficient (TLCO/V_A, DLCO/V_A or KCO). A diffusion disorder, e.g. in lung fibrosis, results in a reduction of TLCO (DLCO) and transfer coefficient (KCO, DLCO/V_A). In contrast, an isolated reduction of TLCO with normal KCO is the result of a reduced lung volume available for diffusion without a barrier to diffusion, e.g. post-pneumonectomy (Figure 6.2). It is important to consider the current haemoglobin (Hb) content because a reduced number of erythrocytes will result in a reduced uptake of carbon monoxide, falsely indicating a diffusion disorder. There are different equations to correct for Hb content; usually they are incorporated into most available modern machines, and one of them is mentioned in Equation 6.1.

EQ Equation 6.1

TLCO Correction for Haemoglobin

$$\text{Men: TLCO}_{Hb} = \text{TLCO}_{measured} \times 1.4Hb/(14.6 - Hb)$$

$$\text{Women: TLCO}_{Hb} = \text{TLCO}_{measured} \times 1.4Hb/(13.4 - Hb)$$

Hb = Haemoglobin, TLCO$_{Hb}$ = TLCO corrected for haemoglobin.

Frequently, when correcting for Hb content, the diffusion disorder 'disappears'. Several situations may result in an abnormally large CO uptake and higher than normal levels of CO-Hb, such as smoking or exposure to CO-producing engines. Therefore, most reliable results are achieved following smoking cessation 24 h prior to the test.

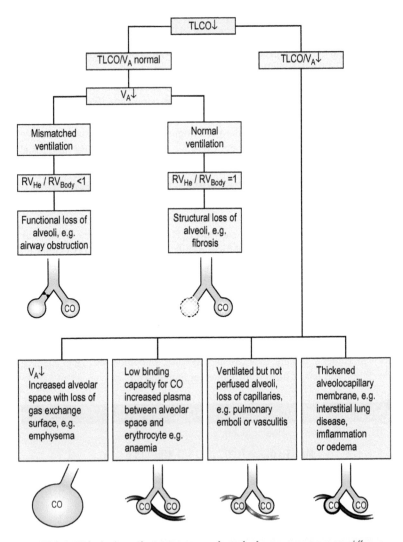

Fig. 6.2 Modified scheme for interpretation of transfer factor measurement in different lung pathologies. RV = residual volume, TLCO = transfer factor for carbon monoxide, V_A = alveolar volume.

Measurements of diffusion capacity facilitate better understanding of lung parenchyma pathophysiology (Figure 6.2). An absolute reduction in TLCO (DLCO) that produces normal results when corrected to the alveolar volume (V_A) suggests a functional or structural loss of alveoli (Figure 6.2). A reduction in TLCO with reduced results relative to the alveolar volume (V_A) suggests a clear decrease in diffusion capacity per alveolar unit (Figure 6.2).

What parameters may influence diffusion capacity?

Diffusion capacity and gas exchange may be influenced not only by atelectasis, alteration of alveolar space and structural loss of alveoli, but also by factors altering the basal membrane, pulmonary vasculature and perfusion. Therefore, diffusion capacity provides important additional information on the function of the lung, in relation to ventilation and perfusion and the air–blood membrane.

As shown in Figure 6.2, measuring the gas transfer may help to differentiate between different causes of pulmonary disease; some typical changes are summarised in Table 6.2.

Table 6.2 Restrictive ventilatory disorders and their influence on lung volumes and gas exchange

Cause	Disease	Lung Function
Pulmonary	Alveolitis, pulmonary embolism, lung fibrosis	$TLC_{body} = TLC_{He}$, TLCO (DLCO) ↓, KCO ↓
Extrapulmonary pleural	Pneumothorax, pleural pathology	$TLC_{body} \geq TLC_{He}$, TLCO (DLCO) ↓, KCO normal
Extrapulmonary thoracic	Obesity, kyphoscoliosis	$TLC_{body} \geq TLC_{He}$, TLCO (DLCO) ↓, KCO normal
Extrapulmonary neuromuscular	Phrenic nerve palsy, motor neuron disease, amyotrophic lateral sclerosis	$TLC_{body} = TLC_{He}$, TLCO (DLCO) ↓, KCO normal

TLC_{body} = TLC measured by body plethysmograph, TLC_{He} = TLC measured by helium dilution method, TLCO (DLCO) = transfer factor for carbon monoxide, Krogh index = KCO.

111

ALVEOLO-CAPILLARY DIFFUSION

The gas transfer may be influenced by several factors that affect diffusion (Figure 6.3):

- Alveolar diffusion distance: increased distance will reduce the number of gas molecules diffusing into the blood by increasing the time they need to reach the lower partial pressure region.

- Alveolo-capillary membrane consisting of alveolar epithelium, interstitial space and capillary endothelium: a thickening of the alveolo-capillary membrane will increase the barrier and resistance between alveolar space and blood, and reduce the number of molecules diffusing per time unit.

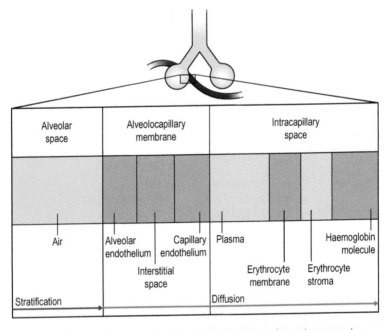

Fig. 6.3 *Diffusion of the oxygen from the alveolar space into the erythrocyte to the haemoglobin, and the anatomical structures that may interact with the diffusion capacity.*

- Plasma: a relatively high (or low) amount of plasma may alter the distance between the erythrocytes and intra-alveolar airspace and influence the amount of molecules diffusing from the higher to the lower partial pressure per time unit.

- Erythrocyte membrane/stroma: theoretically, changes in the erythrocytes' membrane and stroma may interact with diffusion capacity by creating higher or lower resistances.

Understanding the diffusion capacity (TLCO or DLCO) and its component parts is aided by the Roughton and Foster equation (Equation 6.2), which separates the membrane from the reactive conductance.

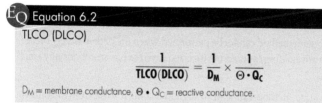

EQ Equation 6.2

TLCO (DLCO)

$$\frac{1}{TLCO(DLCO)} = \frac{1}{D_M} \times \frac{1}{\Theta \cdot Q_C}$$

D_M = membrane conductance, $\Theta \cdot Q_C$ = reactive conductance.

In this model, the membrane conductance reflects the properties from the alveolar epithelium to the interior of the red cells. The reactive conductance reflects the rate of reaction of the gas with haemoglobin (Θ) and the volume of blood in the capillaries (Q_C).

INDICATIONS AND CONTRAINDICATIONS

In certain pulmonary conditions it is important to gain information in addition to standard spirometry, lung volume measurements or blood gas analysis. Some more common indications for diffusion and gas exchange measurement are:

- Diagnosis and follow-up of interstitial lung disease: the gas transfer measurement is important in the diagnostic approach towards interstitial lung disease, as changes in the spirometry, lung volumes, chest X-ray and even blood gas analyses at rest may be small, particularly in early interstitial lung disease.

113

• Diagnosis and follow-up of lung emphysema: as the measurement of gas transfer is very sensitive, although non-specific for chronic obstructive pulmonary disease (COPD), it is a good marker to describe the degree to which oxygen uptake is inhibited in a patient with a hyperinflated chest. It may also help to differentiate between chronic asthma in which diffusion is usually normal, and emphysema. Both TLCO and KCO are closely correlated with emphysema severity, as measured on the CT of the chest.

• Differential diagnosis of other respiratory disorders: early indication of abnormal diffusion is a highly sensitive investigative test; in complex cases, with atypical presentation, it may be a very sensitive and early indicator of various pathologies and may objectively indicate to what extent breathlessness is caused by organic changes.

There are few contraindications to these measurements; however, in certain circumstances, it is important to consider the following before ordering the test:

• The single-breath method cannot be performed when the patient is very breathless (as a breath-holding/apnoea of 10 s is required) or has an abnormally small VC (< 1.5 L).

• The steady-state method can lead to high and almost toxic CO-Hb concentrations and should be avoided in severely hypoxic patients. CO has a high affinity to bind to Hb and toxic levels can only be treated with hyperbaric oxygen, which increases the content of oxygen in solution as the CO-Hb cannot take up any more oxygen.

PITFALLS IN TLCO (DLCO) MEASUREMENTS

Although diffusion measurement is a valuable method, there are common pitfalls that need to be considered when measuring TLCO (DLCO). The breathing manœuvre needs to be accurate, particularly when using the single-breath method, as severe airway obstruction will delay expiration and the washout period (Figure 6.1) and therefore the gas sample will be taken from an unrepresentative gas mix. Similarly, a low vital capacity and a breathless patient may lead to inaccurate measurements. Common mistakes may arise from not correcting for abnormal levels of Hb, as this will affect the binding capacity for CO (Equation 6.1). However, for very low Hb levels, even the correction factors may be naccurate. The steady-state method should not be used in severe degrees of anaemia or haematological abnormalities. It is also worth mentioning that, in smokers, the HbCO is elevated and can influence the measurements significantly. Sometimes, smokers deny that they still smoke when asked by health professionals, and randomly performed HbCO measurements reveal surprising results.

BLOOD GAS ANALYSIS: INTRODUCTION

The overall efficiency of the lung as a gas exchange interface between ambient air and body can best be identified by the arterialised blood. There are different ways to draw blood for this analysis: either it can be taken from an artery, most commonly the radial artery (although the brachial or femoral artery can be used), or it can be drawn from a capillary sample of the hyperaemic earlobe. The blood sample facilitates measurement of paO_2, $paCO_2$ and proton ion concentration (H^+), determining the pH. Other parameters can be derived from those measured. Capillary samples tend to underestimate paO_2 values compared to arterial blood samples, whilst $paCO_2$ and pH are usually almost identical with both forms of analysis. However, for routine measurement, an earlobe blood gas analysis performed by experienced laboratory staff is sufficient, although a representative sample may be difficult to obtain in a patient with shock. The advantage of the earlobe blood gas analysis compared to an arterial sample is that it is easy, accessible, low-risk and minimally invasive.

PARAMETERS DERIVED FROM THE BLOOD GAS ANALYSIS

Arterial paO_2

The partial pressure of oxygen is measured in mmHg or kPa (conversion factor is 7.5; Table 6.5). It is a marker for alveolar gas exchange and is age-dependent.

Oxygen Saturation

The oxygen saturation is directly measured. It is further calculated as oxygen content per oxygen capacity (O_2 content/O_2 capacity), where the content is the amount of oxygen combined with Hb, and the capacity marks the total binding capacity of haemoglobin. It is expressed as a percentage and depends on the partial pressure of oxygen (Figure 6.4).

115

Arterial pH

The pH is the negative decimal logarithm of H^+ ion concentration in the arterial blood. It is regulated by metabolic or respiratory factors. A respiratory acidosis is caused by a pH decrease resulting from $paCO_2$ retention, e.g. due to alveolar hypoventilation, without metabolic compensation. A respiratory alkalosis is caused by an increase in pH resulting from low $paCO_2$ levels due to alveolar hyperventilation without metabolic compensation (acid–base balance, p. 119).

Arterial paCO$_2$

The partial pressure of carbon dioxide ($paCO_2$) is measured in mmHg or kPa and is age-independent. Due to the good diffusion of CO_2, it is a good marker for alveolar ventilation; hypocapnia is derived from alveolar hyperventilation and hypercapnia from alveolar hypoventilation.

Standard Bicarbonate

This refers to HCO_3^- concentration during standard conditions (37°C, 44 mmHg $paCO_2$, full O_2 saturation of the Hb). This parameter (in mmol/L) is calculated from the above parameters.

Base Excess

Base excess (in mmol/L) is calculated from the parameters described above, to summarise the acid–base metabolism. A positive base excess describes an excess of basal equivalents (e.g. in alkalosis) while a negative base excess indicates a lack of bases (e.g. in acidosis).

HOW TO OBTAIN A BLOOD GAS SAMPLE

Blood gases are traditionally taken with a sample either from the radial artery or from an arterialised earlobe, but a sample may be taken from other arteries (e.g. brachial, femoral) as well. When taking the sample from the earlobe, the skin should be prepared so that it becomes hyperaemic (e.g. with cream). After around 10 minutes the cream is removed and a needle is used for a small puncture. The first blood drop should not be used for collection. In addition, the earlobe should not be squeezed, in order to avoid artefactual changes in the test results. The capillary used to collect the blood should be entirely filled with blood to prevent an artefactual air bubble interfering with analysis. The analysis should be performed as soon as possible following sample collection. If a measurement has to be performed later, the probe should be cooled.

GAS EXCHANGE DEFECTS

There are basically two different types of gas exchange defect: type I respiratory failure and type II respiratory failure.

Type I Respiratory Failure

Type I respiratory failure is usually caused by a mismatch between perfusion and ventilation. This leads to hypoxaemia with normal or low $paCO_2$. It is important to consider altitude because paO_2 levels drop physiologically when leaving sea level. At sea level a normal oxygen level is $paO_2 > 10$ kPa (>75 mmHg) and the normal range for $paCO_2$ is 4.67-6.0 kPa (36-44 mmHg, Table 6.4). However, during a commercial aeroplane flight, paO_2 may drop slightly and this needs to be considered prior to boarding. When in doubt whether a patient requires oxygen for a flight, a fitness-to-fly test, breathing F_iO_2 of 15% (equivalent to the effect of cabin conditions at maximum altitude) while monitoring arterial blood gases, may help predict whether patients are at risk while flying and need supplemental in-flight oxygen. This may have important medico-legal implications and should be discussed with the patient before making the booking.

Type II Respiratory Failure

If ventilatory requirements increase, due to either a higher load or a reduced capacity of the respiratory muscles, neural ventilatory drive increases to compensate for increased requirements. Once the neural respiratory drive cannot be adapted or maintained further to sustain increased ventilation over time carbon dioxide (CO_2) will not be exhaled sufficiently leading to CO_2 retention and hypercapnic respiratory failure. Central or thoraco-pulmonary causes of impaired gas exchange can be distinguished by calculating the alveolo-arterial oxygen gradient ($AaDO_2$, Table 6.3; Equation 6.3).

117

Table 6.3 Classification of gas exchange defects using paO₂ and paCO₂ parameters

Gas Exchange Defect	PaO₂	PaCO₂	AaDO₂
Normoxaemia with hypocapnia	n	↓	↑
Type I respiratory failure with normocapnia	↓	n	↑
Type I respiratory failure with hypocapnia	↓	↓	↑
Type II respiratory failure, neuromuscular	↓	↑	n
Type II respiratory failure, cardiac	↓	↑	↑

AaDO₂ = alveolo-arterial difference in oxygen, n = normal, paCO₂ = partial pressure of carbon dioxide, paO₂ = partial pressure of oxygen; ↑ = increased, ↓ = decreased.

CONSIDERATION OF paCO₂ STANDARDISATION

In some cases, hyperventilation can compensate for hypoxaemia. Considering only the paO₂ may in this case falsely imitate normoxaemia. Therefore the paCO₂ level has to be considered for test interpretation as well. This can be achieved by calculating paO₂ according to a standard normal level of paCO₂. For the purpose of using a normal paCO₂ level of 5.3 kPa (40 mmHg), standard equations can be used to correct and standardise the paO₂ level.

ALVEOLO-ARTERIAL PRESSURE GRADIENT (AaDO₂)

The AaDO₂ (Equation 6.3) describes the difference between alveolar and arterial oxygen concentration. In addition to pulmonary disorders, cardiac problems may also result in an increase in the AaDO₂.

EQ Equation 6.3

Alveolo-Arterial Oxygen Gradient (AaDO₂)

$$AaDO_2 = (P_B - P_{H2O}) \times F_iO_2 - (paCO_2/RQ)$$

F_iO_2 = inspired O_2 content (room air = 0.21), P_B = barometric pressure, around 101 kPa (= 758 mmHg) at sea level, P_{H2O} = water saturation of airway gas, around 6.2 kPa (= 46.5 mmHg; fully saturated), $paCO_2$ = partial pressure of arterial CO_2 in kPa or mmHg, RQ = respiratory quotient, usually around 0.8.

The normal range of AaDO₂ increases with age, e.g. 0.2–1.5 kPa (= 1.5–11.3 mmHg) aged 25 years, 1.5–3.0 kPa (= 11.3–22.5 mmHg) aged 75 years.

SHUNT FRACTION

In a patient with hypoxaemia who does not adequately react to supplemental oxygen it may be helpful to define the shunt fraction. This can be important because an arterio-venous shunt can cause oxygen-refractory hypoxaemia. To measure the shunt fraction, the patient needs to breathe 100% oxygen through a full face mask and the capillary oxygen content is measured after 10 minutes. The shunt fraction can then be calculated from standard equations. A reference value for the shunt fraction should be less than 5%. Nuclear methods can also be used for this measurement.

NORMAL PARAMETERS

Hypoxaemia and hypercapnia can be classified into mild, moderate and severe types. However, several national or international societies may use slightly different parameters; thus, the absolute results of a blood gas sample should be interpreted with caution. It is more important to correlate the results of oxygen/carbon dioxide analysis with the acid–base status (pH, BE) of the patient to understand whether changes are compensated for or causing a respiratory or metabolic acidosis or alkalosis. Hypoxia is defined as a paO_2 of less than 8.0 kPa (= 60 mmHg), hypercapnia as a $paCO_2$ above 6.0 kPa (= 45 mmHg). Normal parameters are summarised in Table 6.4.

ACID–BASE BALANCE

The acid–base relationship is important to maintain homeostasis in the body. It can be regulated by metabolic adaptation and ventilation. By excreting H^+ ions

Table 6.4 Reference values for normal parameters in mmHg and kPa

Parameter	Normal Parameters
pH	7.36–7.44
	(H^+ 37–43 nmol/L)
paO_2	> 12 kPa/> 10 kPa in the elderly
	(> 90 mmHg/> 75 mmHg in the elderly)
$paCO_2$	4.67–6.0 kPa
	(36–44 mmHg)
BE	± 3mmol/L

BE = base excess.

through the kidneys and regulating ventilation to influence the $paCO_2$ levels the body attempts to regulate the pH to a range between 7.36 and 7.44. Changes in ventilation may lead to a rise or fall in $paCO_2$. CO_2 is an acid gas which will dissociate with water to H^+ and HCO_3^-. It needs buffering with haemoglobin and plasma proteins. An acute increase in $paCO_2$ may lead to a drop in pH, while lower than normal levels of $paCO_2$ will cause an alkalosis. When chronic elevated levels of $paCO_2$ persist, e.g. in association with hypoventilation, the kidneys try to compensate by retaining bicarbonate. When the bicarbonate level is above the normal level of 25 mmol/L, the difference from the actual measurement is called a positive base excess. In chronic hyperventilation with low levels of $paCO_2$ and higher pH (alkalosis), a negative base excess with less bicarbonate than normal may be observed.

Should there be a metabolic reason for an acidosis (e.g. ketoacidosis), then ventilation may be altered to compensate for the low pH. In a metabolic acidosis, the patient may be hyperventilating (Kussmaul's breathing in ketoacidosis) to eliminate CO_2 and thereby produce a more alkalotic pH. In a metabolic alkalosis, ventilation may decrease in order to cause a more acidotic pH due to CO_2 retention (Table 6.4).

However, the ability to compensate for a condition is more effective with metabolic than respiratory compensatory mechanisms. Thus, metabolic conditions are often only partially compensated for with remaining significant deviations from normal pH, whilst chronic respiratory conditions may be completely corrected by metabolic adaptation. On the other hand, respiratory mechanisms may be altered fast, almost instantaneously, whilst metabolic compensation is a slow process and takes days.

OXYGEN DISSOCIATION CURVE

Under normal conditions, at low oxygen tensions haemoglobin takes up oxygen readily, while at high oxygen tension the opposite is true. Higher temperature, lower pH and more 2,3-diphosphoglycerate (2,3DPG) in the blood are responsible for a shift of the oxygen dissociation curve to the right (Figure 6.4). This means that, with the same amount of oxygen saturation (SpO_2), partial pressure of oxygen in the tissue is lower than with lower temperature, higher pH and less 2,3DPG. This may become important in conditions like sepsis, acute (respiratory) acidosis or cardiac arrest scenarios with patients drowning in icy waters (Figure 6.4). Fetal haemoglobin (HbF) has a higher affinity to bind oxygen and shifts the oxygen dissociation curve to the left.

The partial pressure of oxygen in the blood at which the haemoglobin is 50% saturated is known as the P50. An increased P50 indicates a rightward shift of the

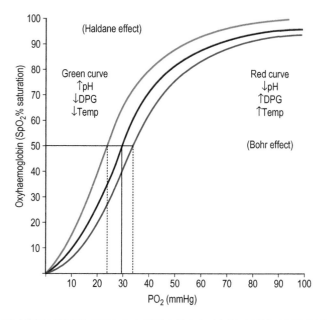

Fig. 6.4 *The S-shaped oxygen dissociation curve (blue line). Blood pH, temperature and 2,3-diphosphoglycerate (2,3DPG) content of the blood can influence and shift the binding curve to either side (red, green and dotted lines), as illustrated by the shift of the P_{50} (paO$_2$ at which oxygen saturation is 50%; see also Haldane and Bohr effects).*

standard curve, which means that a larger partial pressure is necessary to maintain a 50% oxygen saturation. This indicates a decreased affinity. A lower P50 indicates a leftward shift and a higher affinity.

> **? Why is it important to measure SpO$_2$ (%) and paO$_2$ (kPa or mmHg)?**
>
> Due to the non-linear relationship between oxygen saturation and partial pressure in the blood, it is important to have both pieces of information available; large changes in SpO$_2$ can be associated with minimal changes in paO$_2$ and vice versa. As the shift of the oxygen dissocation binding curve is influenced by multiple other factors, measuring only SpO$_2$ may lead to medical staff being dangerously reassured.

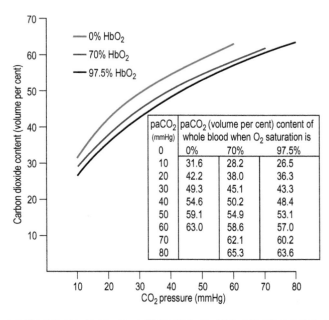

The table in the figure:

paCO$_2$ (mmHg)	paCO$_2$ (volume per cent) content of whole blood when O$_2$ saturation is		
	0%	70%	97.5%
0			
10	31.6	28.2	26.5
20	42.2	38.0	36.3
30	49.3	45.1	43.3
40	54.6	50.2	48.4
50	59.1	54.9	53.1
60	63.0	58.6	57.0
70		62.1	60.2
80		65.3	63.6

Fig. 6.5 The CO$_2$ dissociation curve. The curve is more linear than the one for oxygen and has no maximum plateau.

CARBON DIOXIDE DISSOCIATION CURVE

The CO$_2$ dissociation curve differs from the oxygen dissociation curve in several ways. Firstly, it is more linear and the position of the curve is influenced by the state of oxygenation of the haemoglobin. It has a steeper slope but, more importantly, there is no effective plateau or maximum CO$_2$ content (Figure 6.5).

HALDANE AND BOHR EFFECTS

There is a reciprocal interaction between oxygen and carbon dioxide in the blood. To ease blood gas transport, an increased paCO$_2$ decreases the affinity between haemoglobin and oxygen, the so-called Bohr effect. This allows oxygen to dissociate easier from haemoglobin. On the other hand, a decreased paO$_2$ leads to an increase in carbon dioxide content, the so-called Haldane effect (Figure 6.6). As a consequence, there is improved oxygen uptake in the lung and CO$_2$ elimination from the tissue.

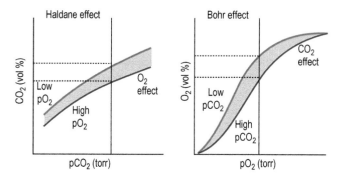

Fig. 6.6 *The Haldane and the Bohr effects, explained by the shift of the carbon dioxide (left) and the oxygen (right) dissociation curves. High levels of oxygen shift the CO_2 dissociation curve to the right, promoting release of CO_2 in the lung, while low oxygen levels, e.g. in the capillaries, stimulate CO_2 uptake in the blood as the curve shifts to the left (Haldane effect). A high CO_2 level in the tissue promotes the discharge of oxygen from the haemoglobin, shifting the oxygen dissociation curve to the right; the opposite is true once the CO_2 level sinks when reaching the lung (this effect is summarised by stating the P_{50}, Bohr effect).*

ALTITUDE AND INSPIRED OXYGEN

Although the percentage of oxygen in inspired air is constant at different altitudes, the fall in atmospheric pressure at higher altitude decreases the partial pressure of inspired oxygen and the driving pressure gradients for gas exchange in the lung. The weight of the air above us is responsible for the atmospheric pressure, which is normally about 100 kPa ($= 750$ mmHg) at sea level.

Atmospheric pressure is the sum of the partial pressures of the constituent gases, oxygen and nitrogen, and also the partial pressure of water vapour 6.3 kPa ($= 47.3$ mmHg) at 37°C.

As oxygen is 21% of dry air, the inspired oxygen pressure (P_iO_2) is $(100-6)$ 94 kPa (705 mmHg) $\times 0.21 = 20$ kPa (150 mmHg) at sea level.

Barometric pressure halves for each 20 000 feet (6000 m) of ascent. At 20 000 feet (6000 m), 21% of the P_iO_2 is $(50-6)$ 44 kPa (330 mmHg) $\times 0.21 = 9$ kPa (67.5 mmHg).

The paO_2 can then be calculated as $paO_2 = 9$ kPa (67.5 mmHg) $-$ $paCO_2$ / $0.8 = 9$ kPa (67.5 mmHg) $-$ 5 kPa (35 mmHg) / $0.8 = 3$ kPa (22.5 mmHg).

123

Therefore, ventilation must be increased at 20 000 feet (6000 m) and a doubling of ventilation would lead to a paO_2 of 6 kPa (= 45 mmHg). However, at the same time, $paCO_2$ would decrease to 2.5 kPa (= 18.8 mmHg). These changes explain the development of Cheyne–Stokes-respiration (Chapter 1) during acute exposure to altitude as the body alternates between hyperventilation to incorporate more oxygen, followed by apnoeas due to a low $paCO_2$ with increase in plasma pH and cerebrospinal fluid (respiratory alkalosis).

During the acclimatisation process there is a gradual increase in red cell volume with erythropoietin stimulation, increased Hb concentration and increased oxygen-carrying capacity of the blood. Hypoxia also leads to an increase in 2,3DPG, which shifts the oxygen dissociation curve to the right, thus favouring unloading of oxygen to the tissue. However, this effect may be counterbalanced by the respiratory alkalosis, which shifts the curve to the left. Eventually HCO_3 content will be reduced as a metabolic compensation (negative base excess) to neutralise the pH.

CONVERSION CHART / paO_2 AND SpO_2 AT A GLANCE

The partial pressure in mmHg is equal to the partial pressure in kPa multiplied by 7.5, while kPa is calculated by dividing mmHg by 7.5. A conversion chart for the different units is provided in Table 6.5.

Table 6.5 Comparison of partial pressures of oxygen, in kPa and mmHg, and oxygen saturation for standard conditions without a shift in the oxygen dissociation curve

kPa	mmHg	SpO_2 (%)
15.0	112	98
10.8	81	96
9.3	66	94
8.4	63	92
7.7	58	90
7.3	55	88
6.8	51	86
6.5	49	84
6.2	47	82
5.9	45	80
5.4	40	70
4.2	31	60
3.5	27	50

SUMMARY

The functional capacity of gas uptake of the lung is reflected in the measurement of diffusion. This measurement is performed by either the single-breath or the steady-state method, using carbon monoxide as a marker in a gas mixture. TLCO (DLCO) describes the total diffusion capacity of the lungs while KCO, as a rate constant, determines the capacity for the given volume. Identifying the diffusion capacity may facilitate differentiation between lung pathologies and is an important marker, particularly in interstitial lung disease or emphysema.

Blood gas analysis identifies the partial pressure of oxygen (paO_2) and carbon dioxide ($paCO_2$). Low levels of oxygen with normal carbon dioxide are considered to constitute type I or hypoxic respiratory failure (mainly $\dot{V}_A/\dot{Q}$ mismatch), usually caused by impaired ventilation. Low levels of oxygen combined with elevated levels of carbon dioxide is consistent with type II or hypercapnic respiratory failure: in other words, hypercapnia due to respiratory pump or controller failure.

Respiratory and metabolic acidosis or alkalosis are characterised by a change in pH. Respiratory conditions are compensated for by slow metabolic changes, while metabolic conditions can impact rapidly on our breathing pattern (hyperventilation) in an attempt to correct the pH.

CHAPTER 7

Basics of Exercise and Respiratory Muscle Testing

KEY POINTS: EXERCISE

- A range of tests is available to assess patients and healthy subjects during exercise. Most common are walking tests such as the 6-minute and the shuttle walking tests. Cardiopulmonary exercise testing (CPET) is the reference method to monitor respiratory, cardiac and metabolic function concurrently and accurately during exercise.
- Anaerobic threshold (AT), endurance workload and maximal oxygen uptake ($\dot{V}O_{2max}$) determine the individual exercise capacity facilitating assessment of chronic cardiopulmonary diseases objectively and monitoring therapeutic effects.
- $\dot{V}O_{2max}$ is an excellent prognostic marker prior to pulmonary surgery.
- Highly specialised equipment, staff requirement, expertise and interpretation of test results limit the availability of CPET and favour simpler exercise measures like the 6-minute walk test.

KEY POINTS: MUSCLE TESTING

- The respiratory muscles can be tested using volitional and non-volitional tests.
- Volitional tests are widely available but only high results exclude weakness reliably. Lower results may reflect poor effort.
- Non-volitional tests (e.g. Twitch P_{di}) are more accurate but require invasive measurement of pressures, expensive equipment and experienced investigators.
- The measurement of seated and supine VC with spirometry may yield important information about respiratory muscle weakness.
- Combining test results of a range of respiratory muscle tests may help to improve accuracy of results.

EXERCISE TESTING: INTRODUCTION

Patients with pulmonary disease may be asymptomatic at rest and cardiopulmonary exercise testing (CPET) can be helpful to unmask pathophysiological conditions in these cases. Specific tests to assess exercise capacity may also provide further information regarding the cause and origin of dyspnoea on exertion, preoperative evaluation (Chapter 8), rehabilitation and disability assessment. There are different options for assessing patients' respiratory function with exercise tests:

1. Walk tests
2. Blood gas analysis during standardised exercise (e.g. treadmill, cycle ergometer)
3. CPET analysis of gases (O_2/CO_2) in inspiration and expiration, and invasive measurements such as cardiac output and blood gases.

Usually, exercise tests are performed in conjunction with dyspnoea scores (e.g. modified Borg score, visual analogue score) to determine the level of breathlessness relative to the workload. Exercise tests are contraindicated in certain conditions, particularly acute ones such as acute coronary syndrome, heart failure, respiratory failure, stroke, uncontrolled hypertension or bleeding. However, indications need to be assessed individually. Exercise tests should be stopped if the patient develops chest pain or severe dyspnoea, feels faint or exhausted, or is at risk of falling. During the test, blood pressure and electrocardiogram (ECG) are monitored for the development of arrhythmias, significant ST elevation or depression, insufficient rise or significant drop in heart rate or blood pressure in case the test needs to be stopped prematurely. The test is generally terminated once the predicted maximal heart rate has been achieved.

WALK TESTS/MINIMAL EXERCISE TESTS

There are several walk tests to assess patients with respiratory disease.

6-Minute Walk Test (6-MWT)

The 6-minute walk test is used to assess severity and to follow up chronic broncho-pulmonary or vascular lung disease, like chronic obstructive pulmonary disease (COPD), interstitial lung disease or pulmonary hypertension. It is also used to test patients with chronic cardiovascular conditions, test efficacy of therapy or follow up after surgery. The patient is asked to walk for 6 minutes as far as possible; standard motivational support can be used. The test should be performed in a corridor according to standard criteria (American Thoracic Society guidelines) with a minimum of 30 m per track. Total walking distance and stops should be recorded. Breathlessness, pulse, saturation and blood pressure are measured immediately prior to and following the test. There is a learning effect when the test is repeated so that a valid measure is usually only recorded when the patient has had more than one test. Although several equations have been reported to predict normal parameters for the total distance, it is difficult to refer to anything other than previously individually recorded test results due to the effect of age, gender, body mass, disease type/severity and abnormal blood gases. However, individual test results and particularly follow-up tests provide useful information about improvement, deterioration or therapeutic effects. The 6-MWT distance also correlates well with quality of life and prognosis (normal range above 400 m in most adults). A minimal clinical important difference in the walking distance has previously been described as a change of more than 54 m, but over the last few years meta-analyses of published data have lowered the threshold to approximately 35 m. However, the test is not appropriate for those patients that are handicapped or unmotivated. Acute sickness may pose a contraindication to any exercise test.

Shuttle Walk Tests

Incremental Shuttle Walk Test (ISWT)

The incremental shuttle walk test was devised in an attempt to standardise the walk test. The patient walks between two cones that are placed 9 m apart in time to a set of bleeps played from a tape or CD. The initial speed is slow but increases with time; the patient has to speed up until the distance between the two cones cannot be covered before the following bleep. The test ends when the patient is either too breathless or does not reach the cones within the allotted time. The number of shuttles is marked and the distance calculated. The distance can be used to determine the level of cardiopulmonary exercise training intensity.

In order to account for a learning effect, the test should be performed on two different occasions and the best result noted. If performed on the same day, the repeat test should be started after at least 30 minutes' rest. Only standardised instructions from the CD should be used and no further encouragement should be given.

Indications and contraindications for the ISWT and reasons for its termination are similar to those for the 6-MWT, but a CD player is required to play the recorded instructions and bleeps. On repeating the test, a change of 47.5 m indicates that patients with COPD feel 'slightly better', while an improvement of 78.7 m reveals they are 'better'. Although the ISWT is more standardised, the 6-MWT is still more widely accepted.

Endurance Shuttle Walk Test

The endurance shuttle walk test was developed to complement the ISWT and to assess endurance capacity in COPD. For this purpose the maximal speed is first determined using an ISWT and then an endurance shuttle walking test is performed at 75%, 85% or 95% of the maximal ISWT speed around the same course. The results are repeatable and comparable to endurance treadmill tests.

MONITORING VENTILATION DURING EXERCISE

Oxygen demand is increased during exercise and the lung and the heart compensate for this effect by increasing the oxygen uptake ($\dot{V}O_2$). Minute ventilation ($\dot{V}E$) is increased, firstly by taking deeper breaths and later by increasing the

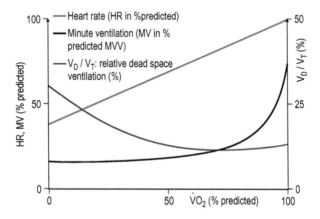

Fig. 7.1 *Schematic display of the relationship between heart rate, minute ventilation and relative dead space ventilation during exercise.* V_D = *deadspace volume,* V_T = *tidal volume,* $\dot{V}O_2$ = *oxygen uptake, MVV = maximal voluntary ventilation.*

respiratory rate. Similarly, the heart rate increases in a linear fashion. $\dot{V}E$ initially increases linearly as well; however, during the course of exercise the increase becomes non-linear with increasing $\dot{V}O_2$ (Figure 7.1).

As ventilation increases during exercise, the relative dead space ventilation (V_D/V_T) decreases. At the same time, the ventilation/perfusion ratio improves by additional recruitment of alveolar volume and pulmonary capillaries, which in turn improves the partial pressure of oxygen (Figure 7.1).

Anaerobic energy consumption is added to aerobic energy expenditure with continued or increasing exercise and this leads to an increase in lactate and more acidotic metabolic conditions. As a consequence, bicarbonate levels fall and the base excess becomes negative.

The minute ventilation is increased to compensate for the metabolic acidotic situation and $paCO_2$ may fall significantly.

In healthy subjects, the heart and not the lung limits exercise capacity!

Walking or cycling exercise tests may be indicated in the diagnostic approach to dyspnoea of unclear origin (pulmonary or cardiac, mixed), gas exchange disorders, assessment of severity and follow-up of pulmonary gas exchange disorders and problems with the respiratory muscle pump, as well as evaluating indications for oxygen therapy.

The patient is most commonly tested on a bicycle ergometer and a standardised incremental protocol should be followed. Some laboratories use a treadmill, which has the advantage of representing everyday function more accurately, but the $\dot{V}O_{2max}$ is higher than on the bicycle ergometer, and it is difficult to quantify external work such as leaning on grab handles or safety bars during the test. However, cycling may be unfamiliar to a lot of patients.

Most commonly, a protocol is used with interval increases of 25 W until task failure. The initial load may be altered according to the patient's health status: a person with severe COPD should start at 0–15 W, while a healthy young subject without respiratory limitation may well start at 50–75 W.

Reasons to stop the exercise may include:

- High heart rate (>220 (beats per minute) − age (years))

- High blood pressure or significant loss of blood pressure

- New changes in the ECG (e.g. extrasystoles, ventricular tachycardia, atrial fibrillation, atrio-ventricular blocks, right or left bundle branch block, Q wave, ST deviation, negative T wave, Q-T prolongation)

- Clinical symptoms (e.g. angina, vertigo, cyanosis, neurological changes, severe dypsnoea, paleness, sweating, drowsiness, ischaemic leg pain, muscle fatigue).

Findings during exercise may include:

- Change in the paO_2: a decrease in paO_2 during exercise might be a marker for diffusion disorder, while an increase in paO_2, when hypoxic at rest, may be observed with ventilation–perfusion mismatch.

- Change in the $paCO_2$: the $paCO_2$ may increase during exercise due to respiratory muscle fatigue or an imbalance in the load-to-capacity ratio of the respiratory muscles with a relatively high load.

- No change in the blood gas analysis: in non-cardiopulmonary exercise limitations (e.g. leg ischaemia), there may be no changes in the blood gases during exercise. However, this may also be the case with a lack of motivation.

- Lactate: the level of lactate indicates the upper level of exercise where metabolic function can compensate for the load imposed by the exercise. Once the anaerobic threshold is crossed, lactate levels will rise and metabolic acidosis will develop.

Blood gas analysis during exercise is a simple and efficient way to assess disease severity, to follow up and to differentiate between pulmonary conditions with altered gas exchange. It is most often used in COPD and interstitial lung disease. It can be helpful in determining oxygen therapy requirements, but this method has increasingly been replaced with walk tests.

Most laboratories use SpO_2 monitoring via pulse oximetry, as it is less invasive than blood gas analysis. Although it has the advantage of not being invasive, it is clearly less accurate than blood gas measurements (Chapter 6). It is important to remember that there are differences in the accuracy of commercially available oximeters and the probes used (e.g. earlobe or finger probe).

 Why do we need cardiopulmonary exercise testing?

Exercise tolerance in cardiopulmonary disease is often low and not predicted by resting measurements. Cardiopulmonary disease is often accompanied by abnormal ventilatory, gas exchange, cardiovascular, limb muscle and acid–base responses to exercise.

CARDIOPULMONARY EXERCISE TESTING (CPET/SPIRO-ERGOMETRY)

Spiro-ergometry incorporates the simultaneous analysis of cardiac, respiratory and metabolic data during exercise, usually on a bicycle ergometer, in order to diagnose cardiopulmonary or metabolic disorders accurately (Figure 7.2). Exercise capacity is determined by different factors:

- Respiratory mechanics and neuromuscular control of breathing
- Alveolar gas diffusion
- Pulmonary ventilation–perfusion mismatch and pulmonary circulation

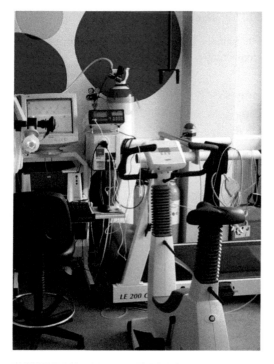

Fig. 7.2 *Equipment for spiro-ergometry and treadmill tests.*

- Quantity and quality of erythrocytes and haemoglobin
- Cardiovascular function and muscular capillaries
- Intracellular energy expenditure, substrates and mitochondrial enzymes
- Deconditioning and lack of fitness, motivation.

It is important to understand the different key parameters that constitute this test, as they indicate whether significant objective limitations are present.

1. Anaerobic threshold (AT): this indicates the point at which the increase in ventilation ($\dot{V}E$) and CO_2 exhalation ($\dot{V}CO_2$) becomes less effective (to eliminate the developing metabolic acidosis) with the start of lactate accumulation. Both $\dot{V}E$ and $\dot{V}CO_2$ increase non-linearly and, because $\dot{V}O_2$ increases linearly, the respiratory quotient ($RQ = \dot{V}CO_2/\dot{V}O_2$) becomes >1. This usually happens at around 50–60% of the maximal workload (W_{max}; Figure 7.3).

2. Workload threshold: this is the point at which the metabolic acidosis can no longer be compensated for and the pH drops.

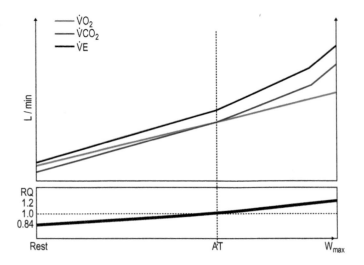

Fig. 7.3 *Ventilation during incremental exercise testing and definition of anaerobic threshold (AT). RQ = respiratory quotient; $\dot{V}CO_2$ = carbon dioxide elimination; $\dot{V}O_2$ = oxygen uptake; W_{max} = maximal workload, $\dot{V}_E$ = minute ventilation.*

3. Maximal oxygen uptake ($\dot{V}O_{2max}$): this is the $\dot{V}O_2$ at maximal workload (W_{max}) just before task failure; pH usually drops to levels of around 7.25, and $\dot{V}E$ is 60–70% of maximal voluntary ventilation (MVV). Predicted values are adjusted according to age, gender and weight (Figure 7.3).

During exercise, airflow is measured via a pneumotachograph, which allows identification of tidal volume (VT), respiratory rate (RR) and $\dot{V}E$. $\dot{V}E$ increases linearly with the workload. In addition, oxygen (O_2) and carbon dioxide (CO_2) are measured during inspiration and expiration, and the difference is used to calculate oxygen extraction and metabolic CO_2 production. Although this is difficult, volumetric data and air flow may be recorded during exercise to determine certain spirometry manœuvres, such as inspiratory capacity to measure the degree of dynamic hyperinflation.

In addition to these measurements several other parameters are calculated or derived with every breath.

Respiratory Reserve

The Respiratory Reserve is derived as the difference between maximal voluntary ventilation (MVV is approximately 35–40 times FEV_1) and the actual maximal ventilation (MVV $-$ $\dot{V}E_{max}$). Once the respiratory reserve reaches around 20%, ventilatory capacity has been fully utilised.

Oxygen Uptake ($\dot{V}O_2$)

$\dot{V}O_2 = \dot{V}E \times \Delta O_2$ (the change in oxygen concentration between inspiration and expiration); the maximal oxygen uptake ($\dot{V}O_{2max}$) reflects the maximal aerobic capacity. It depends on body mass and is therefore usually better expressed as $\dot{V}O_{2max}$/kg or standardised to reference equations, as $\dot{V}O_{2max}$ %predicted, which is independent of age and gender. $\dot{V}O_{2max}$ is closely related to disease prognosis and quality of life in cardiopulmonary disease. The slope ($\dot{V}O_2$/Workload (W); usually around 10 mL/W) indicates aerobic capacity and is higher in trained athletes.

Carbon Dioxide Elimination ($\dot{V}CO_2$)

$\dot{V}CO_2 = \dot{V}E \times \Delta CO_2$; carbon dioxide is eliminated to keep the $paCO_2$ and the pH stable. Increases in $\dot{V}CO_2$ run in parallel to those of $\dot{V}E$; it rises more proportionally than $\dot{V}O_2$, which leads to an increase in RQ as exercise progresses. Once the anaerobic threshold is reached, lactate concentration increases. This is buffered by bicarbonates, further increasing CO_2 production, and $\dot{V}E$ and $\dot{V}CO_2$ eventually increase exponentially (Figure 7.3).

Respiratory Quotient (RQ) or Respiratory Exchange Ratio (RER)

RER $(RQ) = \dot{V}CO_2/\dot{V}O_2$; the respiratory quotient at rest is around 0.84 and is predominantly influenced by metabolic utilisation of fatty acids. During exercise, utilisation of glucose increases until it reaches the anaerobic threshold, when it is 100% ($RQ = 1$). Further increase of the RQ above 1.0 is caused by lactate accumulation. An RQ above 1.0 indicates the full metabolic capacity.

Dead Space Ventilation (V_D)

Dead space ventilation is defined as the amount of air that cannot participate in gas exchange. V_D/V_T estimates a relative contribution of dead space ventilation to each tidal volume (Chapter 1).

Oxygen Pulse ($\dot{V}O_2$/Heart Rate (HR))

This is a marker for reduced cardiac function and indicates low ejection fraction, anaemia or disturbed oxygenation. An early plateau is reached during exercise due to cardiac limitation. Oxygen pulse broadly reflects stroke volume. A low O_2 pulse and a flat response mean that reserves of stroke volume and tissue O_2 extraction are exhausted.

Other Parameters

Other, less specific parameters measured during spiro-ergometry may include ECG, pulse, blood pressure, SpO_2, arterial blood gas analysis and the flow–volume curve. These data provide valuable information for exercise termination and monitoring of the patient.

Indications for CPET

CPET is indicated to evaluate exercise capacity in healthy subjects (e.g. athletes) and disease. It allows the clinician to describe severity, to follow up cardiopulmonary limitations and to control therapy effects. It is an important tool in the assessment of workload capacity (e.g. occupational health) and a useful preoperative investigation to assess risk (Figure 8.4; Chapter 8). It also helps elucidate the aetiology of breathlessness.

Equipment

The investigation requires certain equipment. The patient sits on an electronic bike, wearing a full-face mask connected to a pneumotachograph and an O_2/CO_2 sensor. Blood gas analyser, ECG monitoring and blood pressure measurement must be available. All data are collected with an integrating computer for real-time calculation and simultaneous graphic display of all measured and derived parameters. A crash trolley, including a defibrillator, must be available for all exercise tests and rooms must be kept accessible for emergency teams.

Procedure

An initial pulmonary function test can help to determine the default settings for the exercise protocol. However, most commonly, patients cycle at a steady rate of 50–60/min and workload is increased by +25 W every 2 minutes. A submaximal workload of around 75% of the maximal heart rate is what most patient with disease can attain. In young patients or athletes, the incremental protocol can be run until reaching $\dot{V}O_{2max}$. The load can also be increased by 25–50 W every 4–5 minutes to reach steady state. At the end of each level, blood gases should be taken.

Interpretation of Results

In heart failure, the anaerobic threshold and the oxygen pulse are low. In relation to the observed $\dot{V}O_{2max}$, there is a relatively high oxygen pulse with an early plateau. In pulmonary hypertension, there is an insufficient increase in $\dot{V}O_2$ during exercise and there is a low anaerobic threshold. Respiratory limitation can be diagnosed when $\dot{V}O_{2max}$ is low, with $\dot{V}E$ reaching the normal predetermined threshold in the presence of a submaximal heart rate. In restrictive disease, $\dot{V}E$ reaches an early plateau, respiratory rate increases inadequately and the Flow–Volume curve reveals flow restriction. In obstructive lung disease, there is a slow $\dot{V}O_2$ increase, and $\dot{V}O_{2max}$ and MVV are reduced. The results improve after beta-agonist inhalation and typical changes can be observed in the Flow–Volume curve. The obese patient may have a normal $\dot{V}O_{2max}$ and anaerobic threshold, but $\dot{V}O_2$ is high for the achieved workload. In this scenario all recorded parameters are normal but still there is task failure with insufficient motivation. All of these results are usually visualised on a nine-plot graph that is updated in real time with the computer data; the experienced investigator can recognise stereotypical slope patterns identifying abnormal function.

Why is it important to motivate the patient to maximal effort?

The validity of spiro-ergometry results are directly dependent on the fact that the patient reaches maximal workload, as abnormal characteristics, e.g. in the slopes, become more obvious when the patient reaches true physical exercise limitation. If the test is terminated prematurely, the recordings may be very similar to those of a normal subject, as the cardiopulmonary system has not been tested to its limit.

 Which CPET parameter should we look at first?

Parameters can be grouped into two major categories:
- 1. oxygen uptake ($\dot{V}O_2$)-related parameters
- 2. ventilation ($\dot{V}E$)-related parameters.

These two groups analyse two different but interrelated aspects of exercise performance.

SUMMARY: EXERCISE TESTS

Exercise tests are an important tool for assessing cardiopulmonary exercise capacity, differentiating between specific limitations, explaining symptoms such as dyspnoea, patient follow-up, assessing healthy subjects (e.g. athletes) and monitoring the effect of therapy. A range of different tests are available; simple walking tests that can be performed anywhere, treadmill and ergometer tests, and standardised spiro-ergometry which requires special equipment and expertise.

RESPIRATORY MUSCLE TESTS: INTRODUCTION

The respiratory muscles are an important part of the respiratory system. Normal respiratory muscle function is needed for sufficient ventilation. Weakness of the respiratory muscles eventually results in respiratory failure. Weakness can be caused by neurologic (e.g. stroke, neuropathies), neuromuscular (e.g. myotonia gravis, Lambert–Eaton syndrome) or muscular (e.g. myopathies, metabolic diseases) disorders. Tests of respiratory muscle strength, in particular the diaphragm, are therefore an integral part of the approach to certain patients, e.g. those with amyotrophic lateral sclerosis (motor neurone disease).

Contraction of the respiratory muscles causes pressure gradients between anatomical compartments. These pressures can be measured and quantified inside the body. A variety of tests have been developed over the years to assess inspiratory and expiratory respiratory muscle function non-invasively or invasively, volitionally or non-volitionally.

VOLITIONAL TESTS OF INSPIRATORY MUSCLE STRENGTH

Volitional tests of inspiratory muscle strength ('explosive') are maximum static inspiratory mouth pressure (PI_{max}) and maximum sniff tests. They are easy to perform and widely available. However, they rely on patient effort and therefore may not diagnose weakness accurately. Only high normal values reliably exclude muscle weakness.

The result of volitional manœuvres depends on the lung volume at which they are performed. Whilst maximal inspiratory pressure at the mouth approximates to '0' at total lung capacity, it increases with lower lung volumes. Therefore, PI_{max} is most commonly measured at functional residual capacity (FRC) or residual volume (RV). The disadvantage of volitional tests of muscle strength is that they are poorly standardised with change of FRC.

Maximal Inspiratory Pressure (PI_{max})

Maximum inspiratory pressures can be measured from FRC or from RV in a standard way, with the patient seated, wearing a nose clip and using a flanged or round mouthpiece. Repeated efforts are needed until consistent results are achieved and the numerically largest (negative) pressure is noted. The average pressure can be measured over 1 s; alternatively, peak pressure can be noted (Figure 7.4).

Sniff Nasal Pressure (Sniff P_{nasal})

A plug is used to obstruct one nostril and connected to a pressure transducer. At least 5–10 maximal sniffs need to be performed until a consistent value of sniff nasal pressure is reached; the highest numerical (negative) pressure is taken. There is a close relationship between sniff P_{nasal} and sniff P_{oes} ($r = 0.99$) in normal

139

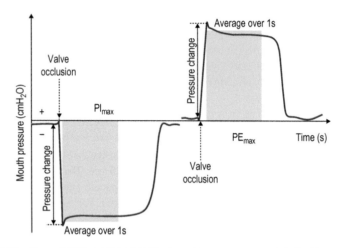

Fig. 7.4 Schematic PI_{max} manœuvre, measured from FRC (left), and PE_{max} manœuvre, measured from TLC (right), following airway occlusion. A maximal effort is made to breathe in (PI_{max}) or blow out (PE_{max}) against the occluded airway and mouth pressure is noted. Either the maximal pressure amplitude or the average of the pressure over 1 s can be noted; it is therefore important to describe the method used.

subjects without nasal obstruction. The ratio of sniff P_{nasal} to sniff P_{oes} is on average 0.91 (Figure 7.5).

Sniff Oesophageal Pressure (Sniff Poes)

Balloon catheters for the measurement of pressure, lubricated with lidocaine (2%) gel, for example, are introduced via one nostril into the oesophagus. Sniff manœuvres are then performed with the patient seated and the balloon catheters in place. At least 5–10 maximal sniffs must be measured; the largest numerical (negative) pressure is noted (Figure 7.5).

Sniff Transdiaphragmatic Pressure (Sniff P_{di})

Pressure catheters are placed in oesophagus and stomach (see sniff P_{oes}) and maximal sniff manœuvres performed as described above. The highest numerical pressure of 5–10 consistent sniffs is taken. Transdiaphragmatic pressure (P_{di}) is derived by calculating the difference between P_{oes} and P_{gas} ($P_{di} = P_{gas} - P_{oes}$; Figure 7.5).

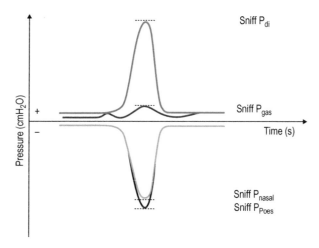

Fig. 7.5 *Pressure recordings during sniff manœuvre. The oesophageal pressure (P_{oes}, blue) is most negative, nasal pressure (P_{nasal}, yellow) is approximately 90% of P_{oes}, and gastric pressure (P_{gas}, red) is a small positive deflection caused by the descending diaphragm squeezing the abdominal content. The transdiaphragmatic pressure (P_{di}, green) is the pressure gradient between oesophageal and abdominal pressures ($P_{di} = P_{gas} - P_{oes}$).*

VOLITIONAL TESTS OF EXPIRATORY MUSCLE STRENGTH

There are two established volitional tests of expiratory muscle strength: maximum static expiratory mouth pressure (PE_{max}) and maximum cough gastric pressure measurement (Cough P_{gas}).

Maximal Expiratory Pressure (PE_{max})

Maximum expiratory mouth pressure is measured from total lung capacity in the standard way, with the patient seated, wearing a nose clip and using a flanged or round mouthpiece. Repeated efforts are made, until consistent results are achieved; the numerically largest pressure averaged over 1 s is measured or, alternatively, peak pressure is noted (Figure 7.4). Mouth pressures can be measured using a simple manometer.

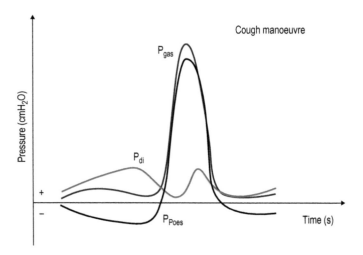

Fig. 7.6 *Pressure recordings during a maximal cough manœuvre. Gastric pressure is highest (P_{gas}, red); the diaphragm is relaxed (low P_{di}, green) and therefore abdominal pressure is transmitted into the chest (P_{oes}, blue).*

Cough Gastric Pressure (Cough P_{gas})

A gastric pressure balloon is positioned as described above (see sniff P_{oes} and P_{di}). The cough manœuvre is performed with the patient seated and wearing a nose clip. Coughs are repeated at least 5–10 times, until consistent measurements are achieved. The numerically highest value is taken, measuring from relaxed end-expiratory baseline gastric pressure to peak pressure during the cough (Figure 7.6).

NON-VOLITIONAL TESTS OF DIAPHRAGM STRENGTH

The origins of non-volitional tests of diaphragmatic strength date back to the 19th century. Duchenne discovered that the diaphragm contracts with electrical stimulation of the phrenic nerves. However, electrical stimulation can be painful and the precise location of the phrenic nerve requires skill to ascertain. In addition, anatomical variations in short or obese necks can make it difficult to achieve satisfactory results and artefactual measurements due to twitch potentiation caused by pain and anxiety have been described.

The development of magnetic nerve stimulation has provided an alternative to electrical stimulation. A rapid change in a magnetic field leads to the induction of an electric current, according to the physical law first described by Faraday. Such electric current leads to the depolarisation of neural structures. In contrast to direct electrical stimulation, this technique generates magnetic fields with deep tissue penetration, avoiding high and irritating currents at the skin that cause pain. Insulated, appropriately shaped coils can be used to stimulate a wide range of nerves (Figure 7.7). The method is reproducible, but the less precise focus in the neck may activate shoulder, neck and upper thoracic nerves and muscles.

Twitch Transdiaphragmatic Pressure (Twitch P_{di})

Twitch transdiaphragmatic pressure is measured following magnetic (or electrical) stimulation of the phrenic nerves, via a unilateral or bilateral anterolateral approach at FRC. The patient is seated, wearing a nose clip, and the mouth is

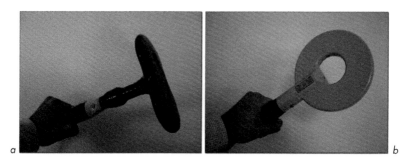

Fig. 7.7 Coils used for magnetic neural stimulation when connected to a magnetic stimulator. **(a)** A figure-of-eight coil, which can be used for unilateral (UAMPS) or bilateral anterolateral magnetic phrenic nerve stimulation (BAMPS); **(b)** The circular coil is used for cervical stimulation or Twitch T_{10}.

143

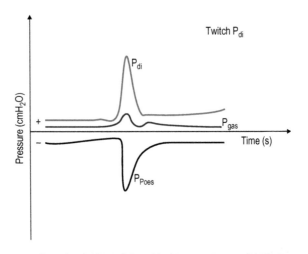

Fig. 7.8 *Recording of oesophageal (P$_{oes}$, blue), gastric (P$_{gas}$, red) and transdiaphragmatic (P$_{di}$, green) pressures following magnetic stimulation of the phrenic nerves.*

closed. Magnetic coils (Figure 7.7) connected to a magnetic stimulator are used; after achieving a supramaximal stimulus, at least five consistent twitches are recorded and the average twitch P$_{di}$ is calculated (Figure 7.8).

NON-VOLITIONAL TESTS OF EXPIRATORY MUSCLE STRENGTH

Twitch T10 Gastric Pressure (Twitch T10)

Gastric pressure is measured after positioning of a pressure balloon, as described above, and magnetic stimulation of the thoracic nerve roots is performed with a circular coil placed with its centre over the 10th thoracic vertebra in the mid-line (Figure 7.7). The manœuvre is undertaken at FRC, with the patient seated, wearing a nose clip, and the mouth closed. Twitches are repeated at least 5–10 times, until consistent measurements are obtained, and an average twitch

T10 is calculated. Twitch T10 is not supramaximal but has been shown to be reproducible.

 Why is it important to have different muscle tests available?

Most available tests of inspiratory muscle strength are volitional and those test results depend on effort and manœuvre. Someone who does not try very hard may have a low PI_{max} result, while a person with an occluded nose may have a low sniff P_{nasal}. In both cases an invasive measurement (e.g. sniff P_{oes}) or a non-volitional test (e.g. twitch P_{di}) may reveal normal inspiratory muscle strength because, in tests of muscle strength, the highest score indicates the real strength. Having a range of tests available to choose from is important to perform further investigations and complete the diagnostic approach in more complicated patients.

ELECTROMYOGRAM (EMG) OF THE RESPIRATORY MUSCLES AND NEURAL RESPIRATORY DRIVE

The recording of electrical activity from muscle tissue is called electromyography. It provides information about the functioning of motor units. This can allow the identification and localisation of pathological processes. Various techniques exist to register the EMG: intracellular, extracellular but intramuscular, and extramuscular. Intramuscular needle electrodes can be unipolar, bipolar or multi-electrode. Surface electrodes come in different forms (patches, plates of silver or stainless steel). Surface electrodes require conductive jelly and need to be fixed to the surface (adhesive disc, glue). Electrodes can also be mounted on catheters to reach inner organs (unipolar, bipolar, multi-electrode).

There is usually no spontaneous activity in healthy skeletal muscle, and background noise is a sign of incomplete relaxation. In neuromuscular disease, there can be spontaneous activity, known as fibrillation, which is most prominent in denervated muscle. The activation of motor units results in the recording of motor unit action potentials in the EMG. With stronger contraction of the muscle, the spontaneous EMG summates the activity of multiple motor unit action potentials, resulting in a crescendo–decrescendo pattern (Figures 7.9 and 7.10).

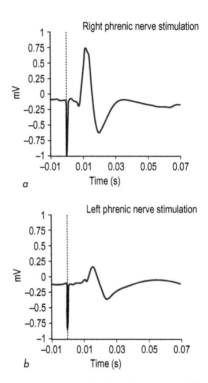

Fig. 7.9 *Compound muscle action potential (CMAP) of the diaphragm, measured with a transoesophageal multi-pair electrode using unilateral anterolateral magnetic phrenic nerve stimulation (UAMPS). (a) The right phrenic nerve shows a normal latency and amplitude; (b) The left phrenic nerve reveals a diminished response with prolonged latency in a patient with left-sided neuralgic amyotrophy. The initial spike is the stimulation artefact.*

Electromyogram of the Diaphragm

The electrical activity of the diaphragm is a surrogate marker for neural respiratory output to the respiratory muscle pump. The diaphragm EMG can provide information about function, activation, treatment effect and neural respiratory drive.

There are different ways to access the diaphragm and record the EMG: noninvasively with surface electrodes, with needles, and with transoesophageal catheters. Best clinical results have been based on the use of transoesophageal multi-pair electrodes recording the diaphragm EMG. This approach is less affected by obesity, power-line artefacts and cross-talk; it is more reproducible than surface EMG and less invasive, and thus is more feasible than needle EMG.

A transoesophageal catheter picks up the signal from the crural part of the diaphragm, whilst the surface EMG records activity from the costal part. However, electrical activity of costal and crural parts of the diaphragm correlates closely. When first developed almost half a century ago, oesophageal catheters had only two electrodes. Movement artefacts made it necessary to develop multi-pair electrode catheters that record the electrical signal over a longer distance. PI_{max}, maximum sniff, TLC and MVV manœuvres have been shown to produce maximal or close to maximal activation of the diaphragm.

The spontaneous signal of the diaphragm EMG at the electrically active region can be calculated as the root-mean-square (rectified) of the raw data and expressed as percent of maximum activity. The advantage of transforming the raw data into percent of maximum activity is that test results are comparable between occasions and between individuals, facilitating follow-up of individuals and group and disease comparisons. Besides the recording of spontaneous EMG activity during breathing, it is possible to record the compound muscle actionpotential (CMAP; Figure 7.9) following electric or magnetic phrenic nerve stimulation. Amplitude and latency of the CMAP allow the diagnosis of phrenic nerve and diaphragm abnormalities and correlate well with the diaphragm EMG during maximum spontaneous activity (Figure 7.10).

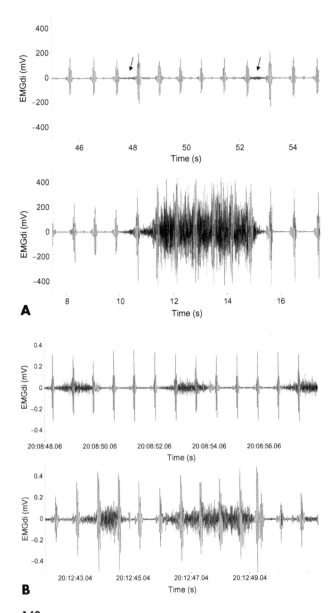

Fig. 7.10, (A) Upper two panels *Periods of spontaneous diaphragm electromyography, recorded from the optimal electrode pair of an oesophageal multi-pair electrode; spikes indicate ECG artefact. Upper panel: spontaneous breathing, seated, in a young healthy subject. Lower panel: TLC manœuvre in the same normal subject, seated.*

*(B) **Lower two panels** Upper panel: Spontaneous breathing in patient with neuromuscular disease, seated. Lower panel: TLC manœuvre in the same subject, seated.*

Inspiratory activity in the normal subject is just visible and is indicated by the two arrows. Note that in the normal subject the resting EMG is a small proportion of TLC manœuvre signal. In contrast, the neuromuscular patient has a reduced TLC manœuvre signal and the resting breathing EMG is significantly increased, reflecting an increased load-to-capacity ratio of the respiratory muscles.

SUMMARY: RESPIRATORY MUSCLE TESTING

There are various tests of respiratory muscle strength and each has its advantages. The most useful assessment of the respiratory muscles starts with non-invasive estimations. Such tests are easy to perform and high values essentially exclude severe respiratory muscle weakness. However, low values obtained from volitional tests do not necessarily confirm weakness, but might be caused by poor effort. More specific for diaphragmatic strength evaluation is the measurement of transdiaphragmatic pressure (P_{di}). For such measurement, gastric and oesophageal balloon catheters are needed. However, all these manœuvres are volitional and only high values can exclude weakness. To confirm weakness non-volitional tests of diaphragm strength are therefore useful. Magnetic stimulation of the phrenic nerves with the simultaneous measurement of P_{di} allows the function of each hemidiaphragm to be tested independently of patient effort. However, the measurement of twitch P_{di} requires expensive equipment and the appropriate expertise. The difference between seated and supine vital capacity (normally less than 10%) may provide further information in neuromuscular disease. A combination of tests to increase diagnostic precision can help support or revise a diagnosis of muscle weakness.

CHAPTER 8

Preoperative Evaluation

KEY POINTS

- A stepwise approach to preoperative evaluation should be adopted.
- Initial assessment should comprise a thorough clinical evaluation.
- If significant abnormalities are detected in the respiratory assessment, then further evaluation should include lung function testing and, depending on the degree of impairment and type of surgery contemplated, exercise testing.
- If significant abnormalities are detected in the cardiac assessment, further evaluation should include exercise electrocardiography and, depending on the cardiac pathology, echocardiography.
- For elective procedures, medical management of the patient should be optimised prior to surgery.

INTRODUCTION

Many patients with a variety of medical problems become candidates for surgery during the course of their life. In this case, the risk of surgery must be balanced against the potential benefit. Although the main risks of surgery are of pulmonary and cardiac origin, other potential complications must always be considered and may include the conditions listed in Box 8.1.

What happens to the lung during anaesthesia?

Frequently, areas of the lung are hypoventilated during anaesthesia. Reduced movement and change of posture promote the development of atelectasis (collapse of one or more anatomical units of the lung).

Box 8.1 Main risks of surgery

Pulmonary
- Pneumonia/atelectasis
- Respiratory failure/mechanical ventilation
- Pulmonary thromboembolism

Cardiovascular
- Congestive heart failure
- Arrhythmias
- Ischaemia/myocardial Infarction
- Hypotension/hypertension

Neurological
- Stroke
- Psychosis

Infection
- Sepsis
- Wound
- Lines

Gastrointestinal (GI)
- GI bleeding
- Ileus
- Cholecystitis

Renal
- Acute renal failure

Metabolic
- Diabetes mellitus
- Porphyria
- Myasthenia gravis

Atelectasis

Atelectasis of a lobule, segment, lobe or entire lung may occur during anaesthesia and invasive ventilation. It has been observed during anaesthesia using assisted spontaneous breathing and during muscle paralysis. Atelectasis occurs regardless of intravenous or inhalational anaesthetics. The occurrence of postoperative atelectasis correlates with preoperative smoking, body weight or body mass index.

Obese patients are more likely to develop larger atelectatic areas than lean subjects. There is a good correlation between the amount of atelectasis and pulmonary shunt, as measured by the multiple inert gas elimination technique (Chapter 6).

Three possible mechanisms may result in lung atelectasis (Figure 8.1):
1. Compression
2. Gas resorption
3. Changes in the consistency of surfactant.

Compression Atelectasis

Compression atelectasis occurs when the transmural pressure distending the alveolus is reduced to such a level that the alveolus collapses. The diaphragm separates the intrathoracic and abdominal cavities and, when active, permits different pressures in the abdomen and chest with the development of a

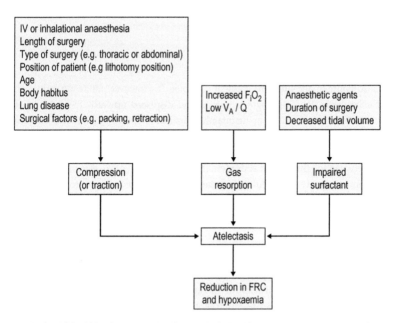

Fig. 8.1 Schematic mechanism of atelectasis formation.

153

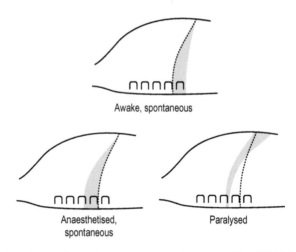

Awake, spontaneous

Anaesthetised,
spontaneous

Paralysed

Fig. 8.2 *Diaphragmatic movement when supine during spontaneous awake breathing and different types of anaesthesia. The grey-shaded area indicates the position of the diaphragm, while the dotted line indicates its physiological upper limit when awake and spontaneously breathing.*

transdiaphragmatic pressure gradient (Chapter 7). However, following induction of anaesthesia, the diaphragm is relaxed and displaced upwards (cephalad) and is therefore less effective in maintaining distinct pressures in the two cavities (Figure 8.2).

As the diaphragm no longer maintains a transdiaphragmatic pressure gradient between the thorax and abdomen, the abdominal pressure is transmitted into the thoracic cavity. The result is that the pleural pressure increases to the greatest extent in the dependent lung regions, which may result in compression of the adjacent lung tissue, i.e. compression atelectasis.

Gas Resorption

Atelectasis caused by gas resorption may occur following complete airway occlusion, forming a trapped gas pocket distal to the obstruction. If there is an increase in the fraction of inspired oxygen (F_iO_2), gas uptake by the blood continues while gas inflow is prevented by the blocked airways, and the gas pocket collapses. Under these conditions, the rate of absorption of gas from an unventilated lung area increases with elevation of the F_iO_2.

Surfactant Changes

The stabilising function of surfactant may be depressed by anaesthetic agents such as halothane and chloroform. Mechanical factors like hyperventilation by increased tidal volume, sequential air inflation to total lung capacity, or even a single cycle of increased tidal volume may cause release of surfactant, as has been shown in animal models.

Anaesthesia and surgery may impair mucociliary clearance and ventilatory drive, and may cause pain and muscle weakness. The use of narcotics and a reduced cough reflex may further contribute to an unfavourable and shallow breathing pattern. This leads to postoperative atelectasis, ventilation–perfusion mismatch and, ultimately, hypoxia, and may cause infection and pneumonia. The majority of postoperative complications following lung resection are due to pneumonia.

 What factors should be taken into account when considering surgery?

Patient-Related Factors

- Age
- Weight
- Current smoking status
- Chronic lung disease
- Cardiac risk
- Obstructive sleep apnoea
- Functional dependence and exercise capability

Procedure-Related Factors

- Surgical site
- Duration of surgery
- Anaesthetic technique
- Surgical techniques
- Emergency surgery
- Extent of resection

Laboratory Assessment

- Respiratory function tests
- Serum albumin
- Blood urea nitrogen
- Full blood count, metabolic, hepatic and renal function

PATIENT-RELATED FACTORS

Age

Increasing age, even after adjustment for comorbid conditions, is associated with an increased rate of operative and postoperative complications. Classically, an age above 70 years is regarded as an independent risk. However, patients in a good state of health should not be excluded solely on the basis of their age.

Weight

The risk of perioperative mortality is dependent on weight. Underweight (body mass index (BMI) $< 18.5 \, kg/m^2$) poses the highest risk, followed by morbid obesity (BMI $> 40 \, kg/m^2$), whereas normal weight and mild to moderate obesity (BMI $18.6–39.9 \, kg/m^2$) seem to carry no increased risk level.

Wound infections are more common in underweight and all obese patient groups, the incidence of superficial wound infection increasing progressively with the BMI.

A reduced BMI ($< 18.5 \, kg/m^2$) is associated with:
- Prolonged hospital stay
- Respiratory complications
- Urinary tract infections
- Cerebrovascular accidents.

Elective surgery in patients with severe obesity (BMI $> 40 \, kg/m^2$) has been associated with:
- Prolonged hospital stay
- Greater likelihood of renal failure
- Greater likelihood of prolonged assisted ventilation.

Obesity is associated with comorbidities (risk increases with BMI):
- Diabetes mellitus
- Systemic hypertension
- Atherosclerotic cardiovascular disease
- Deep vein thrombosis
- Obstructive sleep apnoea
- Obesity hypoventilation syndrome

However, in the absence of substantial comorbidity, mildly to moderately obese patients are not at a significantly higher risk of serious adverse outcomes after elective surgery.

In critically injured obese trauma patients requiring emergency surgery, there is a concomitant increase in mortality when compared with a cohort of non-obese patients, and a significant increase in multiple system organ failure.

Current Smoking Status

When active smokers (without overt chronic obstructive pulmonary disease, COPD) are compared to non-smokers, changes in lung morphometry and immune function have been demonstrated. The alveolar macrophage function is impaired and these cells are less metabolically active and less able to release inflammatory mediators, thus impairing the ability to mount an effective response to infection. There is also goblet cell hyperplasia and other structural epithelial abnormalities that affect the volume and composition of mucus, and decrease mucociliary clearance.

Smoking status is a consistent univariate risk factor in most of the published literature for perioperative pulmonary complications, which include respiratory failure, unanticipated intensive care unit admission, pneumonia, airway events during induction (cough, laryngospasm) and increased need for postoperative respiratory therapy or aerosol therapy. The evidence that children exposed to environmental tobacco smoke have a higher risk of perioperative pulmonary complications would suggest that even relatively low-level exposure to smoke may be clinically important. Smoking also affects postoperative wound-related complications, such as dehiscence and infection.

Smoking cessation improves mucociliary function after as little as a few days but appears to be required for at least 8 weeks in order to affect the number of perioperative pulmonary complications positively, which can be helpful in planning for non-emergency surgery.

However, most studies have been unable to identify preoperative smoking status as an independent risk factor for major cardiac events (e.g. myocardial infarction) during and after either cardiac or non-cardiac surgery.

Chronic Lung Disease

Patients with COPD have an increased risk of postoperative pulmonary complications (PPCs). Risk increases around three-fold compared to normal subjects for unselected surgery and five-fold for thoracic or abdominal surgery.

There is little evidence on the incremental risk for PPCs in patients with chronic restrictive lung disease or restrictive physiologic characteristics due to neuromuscular disease or chest wall deformity, such as kyphoscoliosis. However, clinicians may consider such patients as having an increased risk of PPCs.

Evidence suggests that asthma is not a risk factor for PPCs but common sense would dictate that every attempt should be made to achieve good asthma control preoperatively.

Cardiac Risk

In terms of cardiac risk, postoperative mortality is known to be increased more than two-fold in the presence of an abnormal electrocardiogram (ECG). In addition, surgical mortality within 3 months of a previous myocardial infarction is much increased, and remains significantly higher for up to 6 months. Other accepted risk criteria include more than five premature ventricular contractions per minute, rhythm other than sinus, and the presence of premature atrial contractions on preoperative ECG.

Cardiac Risk Index

There are six known risk factors for perioperative cardiovascular morbidity in the general population (revised cardiac risk index, RCRI criteria). The patient is at risk if they have any one of the factors listed in Box 8.2.

Estimating Preoperative Cardiac Risk

Patients with poor exercise tolerance who report poor functional status, as defined by less than 4 MET, and have 1–2 RCRI criteria and those patients who have a history of angina or claudication are generally suitable for non-invasive testing. (MET stands for metabolic equivalent of tasks and is the physiological concept used to quantify the energy cost of physical activities; for example,

Box 8.2 Revised cardiac risk index criteria

1. High-risk surgical procedure, defined as:
   - Thoracic, abdominal, or pelvic vascular (e.g. aorta, renal, mesenteric) surgery
2. Ischaemic heart disease, defined as:
   - History of myocardial infarction
   - History of/current angina
   - Need or use of sublingual nitroglycerin
   - Positive exercise test
   - Q waves on ECG
   - Patients who have undergone percutaneous transluminal coronary angioplasty (PTCA) or coronary-arterial bypass graft (CABG) and who have chest pain presumed to be of ischaemic origin
3. Heart failure, defined as:
   - Left ventricular failure by physical examination
   - History of paroxysmal nocturnal dyspnoea
   - History of pulmonary oedema
   - S3 or bilateral rales on physical examination
   - Pulmonary oedema on chest X-ray
4. Cerebrovascular disease, defined as:
   - History of transient ischaemic attack
   - History of cerebrovascular accident
5. Insulin-dependent diabetes mellitus
6. Chronic renal insufficiency, defined as:
   - Baseline creatinine $\geq$ 176 μmol/L ($\geq$ 2.0 mg/dL)

1 MET is equivalent to the physical activity when sitting and 2 MET is equivalent to slow walking). Pharmacological stress testing should be pursued in such patients. Patients at higher ($>$ 20%) risk according to initial estimates (RCRI $>$ 3) may still have high perioperative risks despite a negative non-invasive study ($>$ 5% post-test probability with negative test).

Identifying Patients with Aortic Stenosis. Clinicians should screen specifically for aortic stenosis during a careful preoperative physical examination. Patients with physical findings consistent with outflow tract obstruction should be referred for echocardiography.

Identifying Patients with Hypertension. Patients should continue antihypertensive medications up to the morning of surgery and resume them, either orally or intravenously, as soon as possible postoperatively. The general consensus is to delay surgery if blood pressure is sustained at 180/110 mmHg or above in patients with cardiovascular disease.

Identifying Patients with Pulmonary Hypertension and Congenital Heart Disease. No data are specific to the perioperative setting; beneficial therapies for chronic conditions are generally recommended.

Identifying Patients with Heart Failure or Arrhythmias. When possible, surgery should be delayed if the heart failure or arrhythmia is unstable, meets the accepted criteria for new interventions, or is likely to represent ischaemic disease.

Echocardiography. Preoperative echocardiography should not be obtained routinely but should be performed when valvular disease, left ventricular dysfunction or pulmonary hypertension is suspected.

Obstructive Sleep Apnoea (OSA)

OSA is a common disorder, which remains undiagnosed in the majority of sufferers. As surgery in these patients is associated with a higher postoperative complication rate, attempts should be made to diagnose the condition preoperatively.

- Tracheal intubation is increasingly difficult, particularly in patients with the more severe type of OSA thought to be related to upper airway abnormalities (see Mallampati index, Chapter 1).

- Airway management difficulties in the immediate postoperative period are more common.

- OSA is thought to result in an increase in substantial surgery-related respiratory or cardiac complications, which is most marked in untreated patients. There may be a 'protective effect' for OSA patients treated with continuous positive airway pressure (CPAP), in that they seem to have a lower rate of complications following surgery than patients not treated with CPAP. In obese

Table 8.1 American Society of Anesthesiologists (ASA) classification to predict postoperative risk

ASA Class	Class Definition	Rate of PPCs by Class (%)
I	A normally healthy patient	1.2
II	A patient with mild systemic disease	5.4
III	A patient with systemic disease that is not incapacitating	11.4
IV	A patient with an incapacitating systemic disease that is a constant threat to life	10.9
V	A moribund patient who is not expected to survive for 24 hours with or without operation	N/A

subjects it is important to consider the possibility of co-existing obesity-hypoventilation syndrome, requiring non-invasive ventilation to avoid perioperative complications.

Functional Dependence and Exercise Capacity

Functional dependence is an important predictor of PPCs. Total dependence is defined as the inability to perform any activities of daily living. Partial dependence is defined as the need for equipment or devices and assistance from another person for some activities of daily living.

ASA Classification

The ASA (American Society of Anesthesiologists) classification (Table 8.1) is:
- A measure of comorbidity
- Proven to predict both postoperative pulmonary and postoperative cardiac complications.

PROCEDURE-RELATED FACTORS

There are various procedure-related factors influencing perioperative risk (Table 8.2). Procedure-related risk factors are as important as patient-related factors in estimating risk for PPCs.

Table 8.2 Procedure-related factors influencing perioperative risk

Factors
Surgical site
Duration of surgery
Anaesthetic technique
Surgical technique
Emergency surgery (increased surgical site infection)
Extent of resection

Surgical Site

The most important general concept determining the risk of surgery is that the further the procedure from the diaphragm, the lower the respiratory complication rate. Pulmonary complications (which are the most frequent cause of postoperative morbidity and mortality) are more common following upper abdominal surgery than lower abdominal surgery.

There is good evidence that the following procedures are related to increased risk for PPCs:

- Aortic aneurysm repair
- Thoracic surgery
- Abdominal surgery (in particular upper abdominal surgery)
- Neurosurgery
- Prolonged surgery
- Head and neck surgery
- Emergency surgery
- Vascular surgery.

Duration of Surgery

Studies that used multivariable analyses found prolonged surgery duration (> 3 h) to be an independent predictor of PPCs (pooled odds ratio (OR) 2.14, confidence internal (CI) 1.33–3.46).

Anaesthetic Technique

Studies have provided estimates for risks related to general anaesthesia as compared to more local approaches (OR 1.83, CI 1.35–2.46). Theoretically, when compared to general anaesthesia, regional or local anaesthesia has the advantage of avoiding the strong stimulus of intubation and postoperative lung function reduction but in the case of COPD, for example, there is little convincing supportive literature. This may be because COPD patients in particular are often unable to lie strictly supine and become progressively uncooperative with worsening gas exchange; sedation is liable to aggravate these problems. It is important to remember that deep anaesthesia is a major prophylactic against bronchoconstriction, in healthy patients as well as in those with COPD.

Intuitively, pre-anaesthetic treatment with salbutamol would be a reasonable recommendation in asthmatic or other potentially problematic patients suffering from chronic airflow obstruction.

High thoracic epidural anaesthesia (TEA) alone, without intubation, has been performed for a variety of operations. Postoperative pain, especially after thoracic surgery, is a main cause of decreased tidal volumes, resulting in hypoventilation, the formation of atelectasis and pneumonia. Therefore, a combination of TEA and general anaesthesia is widely preferred, particularly in high-risk pulmonary patients. Various studies have shown the beneficial effects of TEA on postoperative pain management, the restoration of lung function and accelerated recovery in thoracic and upper abdominal surgery. Neural sympathetic blockade has also been effective in decreasing the rate of postoperative cardiac complications.

Surgical Techniques

Open thoracotomy and laparotomy are the most established approaches for thoracic and abdominal surgery respectively and are frequently preferred to endoscopic operations, as they offer a better view of the extent of malignancy and better control of bleeding. However, less invasive thoracoscopic and laparoscopic techniques are increasingly utilised, particularly in less complicated cases. Thoracoscopic lobectomy is applicable to a spectrum of malignant and benign pulmonary diseases and is associated with a low perioperative morbidity and mortality rate. Survival rates are comparable and may even be superior to those for lobectomy performed by thoracotomy. Video-assisted thoracoscopic surgery (VATS) for lobectomy in cases of stage I and II non-small cell lung cancer (NSCLC) is associated with shorter chest tube duration, shorter length of hospital stay and improved survival when compared to thoracotomy. The benefits conferred, compared to open thoracotomy, are derived from the less traumatic approach and include reduced postoperative pain, reduced impairment in respiratory muscle and pulmonary function, reduced cytokine production and improved immuno-surveillance.

In addition, although approximately 10% of VATS patients will need an intraoperative conversion to open thoracotomy, usually to control bleeding or because of unexpected location or extent of tumour, conversion during attempted VATS resection does not prejudice short-term or long-term surgical outcomes.

In terms of abdominal surgery, laparoscopic surgery, as compared to open laparotomy, is associated with a reduction in fever, urinary tract infection, post-operative complications, postoperative pain, number of days in hospital and total cost. Immediate postoperative lung function appears to decline more following open laparotomy but no consistent difference in pulmonary complications has been described in the literature.

Emergency Surgery

In studies reporting multi-variable analyses, emergency surgery was shown to be a predictor of significant PPCs (OR 2.25, CI 1.57–3.11) compared to elective surgery.

Extent of Resection

Mortality depends on the degree of resection; typically, mortality figures for a lobectomy and pneumonectomy are within the range of 0.5–4% and 6–8% respectively.

LABORATORY ASSESSMENT

Respiratory Function Tests

Various factors have contributed to a less stringent approach to the operability criteria for resection over the years; they include early mobilisation, deep breathing, intermittent positive-pressure breathing, incentive spirometry and effective analgesia, which may decrease postoperative complications. In addition, the improvement in modern anaesthetic techniques, more readily available intensive care facilities and the recent development of less invasive surgical procedures have reduced morbidity and mortality. Nevertheless, appropriate patient selection is crucial, particularly for thoracic surgery and especially lung resection surgery, in a predominantly smoking (or ex-smoking) patient population with frequent comorbidities. The two critical issues when considering surgical risk are:

1. the patient's ability to survive the physical stress of the operation itself ('operability') without causing severe pulmonary impairment
2. the amount of lung tissue that can be removed ('resectability').

It is important to remember that, even after the most exhaustive preoperative evaluation, a decision may need to be made intraoperatively to resect more lung than originally envisaged, due to tumour extension that was not known or imaged preoperatively, or unexpected surgical complications. Therefore, the surgeon needs to be well instructed as to the patient's operability in relation to the maximum amount of lung resection that can be contemplated.

Over the years, many physicians have made decisions not to refer certain groups of patients to surgery, based on intuitive feelings regarding patient suitability formed by observing their overall condition, including age, weight and various other parameters. To some extent, this is incorporated into the concept behind the ASA classification of functional dependence (Table 8.1). Most of the literature regarding high-risk thoracic lung resection cases contains prospective and/or retrospective preoperative lung function data and relates the results of these tests to subsequent perioperative morbidity and mortality, whilst attempting to take comorbidities into account.

With regard to lung resection and cardiac surgery, there is a widespread consensus about the importance of assessing preoperative lung function, most specifically by spirometry. The situation is different with candidates for extrathoracic surgery; however, intuitively, there are few physicians who would not at least consider performing spirometry in heavy smokers or patients with known COPD or asthma prior to abdominal (particularly upper abdominal) or even extra-abdominal surgery. Additionally, attempts to optimise preoperative lung function should be made in the presence of significant airway obstruction, for example.

Nevertheless, attempts have been made to use the results of lung function testing as part of preoperative thoracic surgery evaluation. When considering lung resection, the question that must be asked is: 'How much is the area of lung to be resected contributing proportionately to overall lung function?' This is relevant because resection of a lobe or lung that is almost completely infiltrated by tumour may not seriously affect overall postoperative lung function if this part of the lung was no longer contributing significantly to gas exchange.

Lung Function Tests for Perioperative Risk Assessment

In terms of lung resection, early data suggested that absolute spirometric values were more relevant. Spirometry reflects the overall mechanical function of the lungs and thorax. The British Thoracic Society (BTS) have stated that no further respiratory function tests are required for a lobectomy if the post-bronchodilator FEV_1 is > 1.5 L or for a pneumonectomy if the post-bronchodilator FEV_1 is > 2.0 L, provided that there is no evidence of interstitial lung disease or unexpected disability due to shortness of breath.

Frequently, however, the clinician is faced with more limited patients and a crucial decision as to whether or not to refer these patients for surgery. In addition, an FEV_1 of 1.5 L may be close to normal predicted values in the elderly population (Figure 8.3).

More recently, percent predicted values have been shown to be more important. There is a consensus regarding the need for spirometry before thoracic surgery in general, and more specifically before lung resection. An FEV_1 of 80% or more of predicted is considered, from a respiratory point of view, to be sufficient for thoracic non-lung resection surgery. However, in the case of a low FEV_1, an attempt is made to predict postoperative lung function, which aims to take into account the functional contribution of the region to be resected.

The percent predicted postoperative (ppo) FEV_1 is intended to estimate what capacity the patient will be left with following surgery. Although ppo-FEV_1 is fairly accurate in predicting the definitive residual value of FEV_1 3–6 months after surgery, the actual FEV_1 observed in the initial postoperative days, when most complications occur, may be much lower. Nevertheless, the ppo-FEV_1 is the best predictor of complications. Initially, the cut-off point was 40% predicted but, in light of recent serious improvements in perioperative management and surgical techniques, the current suggestion is that it should be lowered to 30% (Chapter 3).

The ppo-FEV_1 should not to be used alone to select patients with lung cancer for lung resection. This is particularly true in patients with moderate to severe COPD, as the ppo-FEV_1 tends to underestimate the functional loss in the early postoperative phase; neither does it appear to be a reliable predictor of complications in COPD patients.

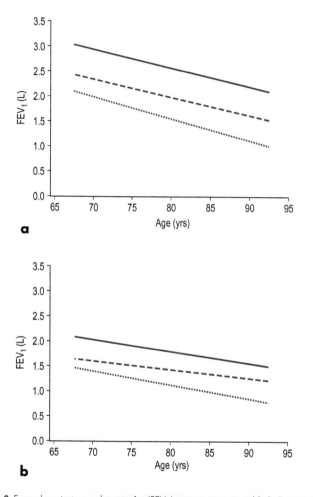

Fig. 8.3 Forced expiratory volume in 1 s (FEV₁) in asymptomatic elderly European never-smokers. **(a)** Males 170 cm in height; **(b)** Females 160 cm in height. Lower 5th percentile and calculated 80% of predicted FEV₁ are shown. The solid line shows predicted values; the dotted line, lower limit of normal; the dashed line, 80% predicted.

However, spirometry measures mechanical properties but not alveolar oxygen exchange. It is therefore important to remember that diffusion is a valuable marker for gas exchange in the assessment of the lung resection candidate in the form of transfer factor (or diffusing capacity) of the lung for carbon monoxide (TLCO or DLCO; Chapter 6). The TLCO (DLCO) decreases following resection of the lung and a low TLCO (DLCO) has been associated with an increased perioperative mortality following lung resection. A ppo-TLCO of less than 40% was previously the accepted cut-off point for an unacceptably high operative risk but, similarly to the ppo-FEV$_1$, the limit has been reduced to 30% predicted as a result of improved perioperative and surgical techniques.

Current guidelines recommend the measurement of diffusion as well as FEV$_1$ in all patients undergoing lung resection surgery.

 How is postoperative lung function calculated?

Percent predicted postoperative (ppo) FEV$_1$ or TLCO calculation, applicable to lobectomy only

Ppo FEV$_1$ (or ppo TLCO%) = measured FEV$_1$% (or measured TLCO%)/100 × ((19 − number of segments resected)/19)

(For segment numbers, see Chapter 1; wedge resection counts as 1 segment.)

Nuclear scintigraphy, applicable to pneumonectomy and lobectomy

Perfusion scintigraphy is a commonly used method to predict ppo parameters pre-pneumonectomy. Both ventilation and perfusion scintigraphy provide a good prediction of postoperative lung function following lobectomy, but in practice, scintigraphy is not widely employed in assessing patients for lobectomy because of the difficulty in interpreting the contribution of individual lobes to overall ventilation or perfusion.

Blood Gas Tensions and Oxygen Saturation at Rest

Hypercapnia does not predict complications by itself, especially if patients can exercise adequately. However, in practice, these patients may be excluded from surgery due to poor spirometry or diffusion measurements, as the finding of hypercapnia usually reflects diffuse respiratory pathology or extrapulmonary causes.

Patients should be further evaluated preoperatively, as they are associated with a higher risk of post-operative complications, if paO_2 is < 8.0 kPa ($= 60$ mmHg) and $paCO_2$ is > 6.0 kPa ($= 45$ mmHg).

Exercise Tests for Resective Lung Surgery

Cardiopulmonary Exercise Testing (CPET). CPET is a comprehensive way of assessing cardiopulmonary systems and systemic oxygen delivery. Maximal exercise testing is incremental and performed on either an exercise bicycle or a treadmill in a controlled environment with real-time monitoring of a variety of cardiac and respiratory parameters. CPET also has the advantage of highlighting the factors that limit exercise (pulmonary, cardiovascular or musculoskeletal), which may help to focus preoperative management on those specific exercise-limiting elements (Chapter 7). The concept is that oxygen uptake, ventilation, carbon dioxide output and blood flow all increase during CPET, and adequate performance on exercise testing is almost certainly reflected in a favourable response to the stress of resective surgery. It has been shown that exercise capacity, expressed as $\dot{V}O_2$ peak (peak oxygen consumption, defined as oxygen uptake at the maximal level of tolerated exercise), is lower in patients that develop postoperative cardiorespiratory complications after lung resection, and appears to be a better predictor of exercise capacity following resective surgery than conventional lung function tests.

- A $\dot{V}O_2$ peak of $> 75\%$ predicted or > 20 mL/kg/min is considered to be the cut-off point for pneumonectomy.
- A $\dot{V}O_2$ peak of $< 30\%$ predicted or < 10 mL/kg/min is considered to be highly risky for any resection.
- A $\dot{V}O_2$ peak cut-off point for lobectomy has not been determined. Therefore, in those cases when the $\dot{V}O_2$ peak is between 30 and 75% predicted or 10–20 mL/kg/min, split function tests are recommended (Table 8.1).

Easy Exercise Tests for Perioperative Risk Assessment. Some centres may not have the facilities to perform CPET and, therefore, a low-technology exercise test may be used as a substitute and screening test (Chapter 7):

- **Stair climbing:** in the past, thoracic surgeons have accepted the climbing of three flights of stairs without interruptions as being satisfactory functional evidence of fitness for lobectomy. Subsequently, systematic studies have been undertaken on large populations of thoracic surgery patients.

169

The conclusions are that, the higher the altitude climbed, the lower the complication rate. Translating this into specifically measurements of height, we see, as with CPET, that below 22 m complication rates are high. In patients who climb less than 12 m, cardiopulmonary complications (two-fold) and overall mortality (thirteen-fold) are higher than in patients who climb more than 22 m. In addition, exercise desaturation $> 4\%$ SpO_2 on a maximal stair-climbing test is associated with an increased postoperative complication rate of 36%. Patients who perform poorly on the stair-climbing test should undergo formal cardiopulmonary exercise testing with measurement of oxygen consumption to optimise their perioperative management.

- **Six-minute walk test:** this is frequently used in clinical respiratory medicine. Both the distance walked along a corridor over a 6-minute period and oxygen saturation before and at the end of the test are recorded (Chapter 7). The parameters associated with a low perioperative mortality are at least 300 m covered during the 6-minute walk, with no more than a 4% reduction in oxygen saturation. Although the distance walked in 6 minutes has been shown to be highly reliable in estimating $\dot{V}O_2$ peak in healthy subjects, COPD and transplant candidates, there is less of a consensus regarding its usefulness in predicting postoperative complications.

- **Shuttle walk test:** this incremental exercise test is useful and readily available. Distance performance on the shuttle walk test correlates significantly with peak oxygen consumption ($\dot{V}O_2$ peak) during treadmill testing (Chapter 7). However, it tends to underestimate exercise capacity at the lower range, compared to $\dot{V}O_2$ peak. Patients who exceed 400 m on the shuttle walk may not need $\dot{V}O_2$ assessment, but if the result is < 400 m a $\dot{V}O_2$ assessment should be performed.

In practice, when considering 'low-technology' exercise testing, the 6-minute walk and the stair-climbing tests are the most frequently used. Thoracic surgeons tend to prefer stair-climbing, whereas chest physicians prefer the 6-minute walk test, despite the fact that the 6-minute walk is not a reliable predictor of a complicated postoperative course. Stair-climbing is a reasonable choice for first-line functional preoperative screening.

Pre-Thoracic Surgery Management Algorithm

The algorithm shown in Figure 8.4 emphasises the importance of a preliminary cardiac assessment. Patients with a low cardiac risk or those who are stable

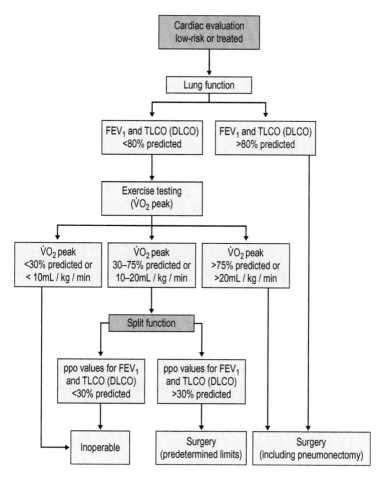

Fig. 8.4 *Algorithm for the management of perioperative risk assessment in patients for thoracic surgery.*

with optimised cardiac treatment can proceed with pulmonary evaluation. Spirometry and diffusion assessment are recommended in all patients. Patients with either an FEV_1 or a TLCO (DLCO) or both below 80% of predicted should ideally undergo formal CPET with peak $\dot{V}O_2$ measurement. However, in practice, many centres may not have the facilities to perform CPET and a low-technology exercise test, preferably a stair-climbing test, may therefore be substituted as a screening test. Should the surgical candidate be unable to climb more than 22 m up the stairs, then formal CPET should be carried out.

Patients with $\dot{V}O_2$ peak < 30% predicted (or < 10 mL/kg/min), or ppo-FEV_1 or ppo-TLCO (ppo-DLCO) or both < 30% predicted values (even if $\dot{V}O_2$ peak is > 30% or > 10 mL/kg/min) are at major risk of perioperative complications for lobectomy or pneumonectomy (Figure 8.4).

If, as a result of comorbidities, patients are unable to perform a satisfactory exercise test, they nevertheless should be regarded as high-risk patients.

The above rules are not absolute criteria but serve as clinical guidance, in that even high-risk patients may be considered for life-saving lung resection under certain circumstances, specifically when patients and surgeons are willing to accept a higher perioperative complication rate to achieve a potential cure, e.g. for lung cancer.

Incidence of and Risk Factors for Pulmonary Complications After Non-Thoracic Surgery

In contrast to thoracic surgery, the indications for routine lung function testing in non-thoracic surgery are not well established. Nevertheless, it makes clinical sense that, in patients with a smoking history and in those with proven COPD, preoperative spirometry should be performed and appropriate therapy should be optimised preoperatively.

Supporting data include the fact that patients with an FEV_1 < 1.2 L undergoing non-thoracic surgery had a 37% incidence rate of PPCs. In patients undergoing non-laparoscopic abdominal surgery, the two best independent predictors of respiratory failure, pneumonia, pleural effusion and pneumothorax were an FEV_1 < 61% of predicted and a paO_2 < 9.3 kPa (70 mmHg). A reduced FEV_1 and FEV_1/FVC ratio were associated with significantly more PPCs. Studies have also shown that the routine use of nasogastric tubes after laparotomy is associated with a higher rate of atelectasis and pneumonia, and current recommendations include only selective and not routine insertion of nasogastric tubes.

Serum Albumin

Low levels of serum albumin are associated with an increased rate of PPCs ranging from 7% to 28% in patients with low serum albumin levels. On the basis of multi-variate analysis, it has been recognised that a serum albumin level of $< 35\,g/L$ is one of the most powerful patient-related risk factors and predictors of risk.

Blood Urea Nitrogen

Serum blood urea nitrogen levels of 7.5 mmol/L or greater ($\geq 21\,mg/dL$) are considered to be a perioperative risk factor. However, the magnitude of the risk seems to be lower than it is for low levels of serum albumin.

SUMMARY

The operability criteria for resection have become less stringent over the years due to the increased use of modern anaesthetic techniques, intensive care facilities and less invasive surgical procedures. However, a stepwise approach, including the history of the patient and assessing risk using lung function and exercise capacity, offers good clinical guidance to minimise perioperative risk.

Index

Printed and bound by CPI Group (UK) Ltd, Croydon, CR0 4YY

03/10/2024

01040847-0002